PENGUIN BOOKS

## *Nee Naw*

Suzi Brent was born in 1977 in a remarkably boring suburb of London. When she was a child she aspired to be a doctor, but soon went off the idea as it looked too much like hard work. In 2004, inspired by the Christmas episode of *Casualty*, she successfully applied to become an Emergency Medical Dispatcher for the London Ambulance Service and has been working there ever since. Suzi is the author of the popular blog *Nee Naw* (www.neenaw.co.uk). This is her first book.

# Nee Naw

*Real-life Dispatches from Ambulance Control*

SUZI BRENT

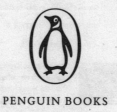

PENGUIN BOOKS

## PENGUIN BOOKS

Published by the Penguin Group

Penguin Books Ltd, 80 Strand, London WC2R 0RL England

Penguin Group (USA) Inc., 375 Hudson Street, New York, New York 10014, USA

Penguin Group (Canada), 90 Eglinton Avenue East, Suite 700, Toronto, Ontario, Canada M4P 2Y3
(a division of Pearson Penguin Canada Inc.)

Penguin Ireland, 25 St Stephen's Green, Dublin 2, Ireland (a division of Penguin Books Ltd)

Penguin Group (Australia), 250 Camberwell Road, Camberwell, Victoria 3124, Australia
(a division of Pearson Australia Group Pty Ltd)

Penguin Books India Pvt Ltd, 11 Community Centre, Panchsheel Park, New Delhi – 110 017, India

Penguin Group (NZ), 67 Apollo Drive, Rosedale, North Shore 0632, New Zealand
(a division of Pearson New Zealand Ltd)

Penguin Books (South Africa) (Pty) Ltd, 24 Sturdee Avenue, Rosebank, Johannesburg 2196, South Africa

Penguin Books Ltd Registered Offices: 80 Strand, London WC2R 0RL, England

www.penguin.com

First published 2010

2

Copyright © Suzi Brent, 2010

Set in Bembo Book MT Std 11/13
Typeset by TexTech International
Printed in Great Britain by Clays Ltd, St Ives plc

A CIP catalogue record for this book is available from the British Library

ISBN: 978-0-141-04437-8

www.greenpenguin.co.uk

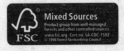

For London's ambulance crews

# Contents

# Prologue

# The London Bombings

'Hello, ambulance. Fire brigade here. We've had reports of an explosion at Liverpool Street underground station. No further details at present. Could we have an ambulance on standby, please?'

'Certainly,' I said, and after exchanging reference numbers with the fire brigade control room, I hung up and settled back down to read that morning's *Metro*, full of happy stories about London's winning Olympic bid. Upstairs, one of the dispatch desks arranged the ambulance without a second thought. It was just before 9 a.m. and there were plenty available. Calls to explosions are not uncommon. Usually they turn out to be nothing – a stink bomb, a gas canister, a small fire at worst.

Then a call taker sitting opposite me took a call from a member of staff at Aldgate East station. I saw her expression change from indifferent to concerned to gobsmacked. She waved a hand in the air to summon a supervisor. A gaggle of call takers peered over her screen to see what the fuss was all about.

'Explosion at location,' read the ticket. 'Walking wounded leaving station with cuts and soot in hair. Delay obtaining info, caller is hysterical.'

Suddenly the call takers began running back to their phones as a Mexican Wave of activity broke out. Similar calls came in from Aldgate, King's Cross and Russell Square. Confusion reigned: where was this incident? Had a caller given the wrong station name in their panic? Or were there two separate incidents? London Underground informed us that they believed a 'power surge' was responsible for the explosions, and that there had indeed been at least two of them.

Quickly, a manager declared a major incident and some of the more experienced members of staff donned fluorescent yellow jackets and went out to the incident control room. The dispatch desks went crazy. The resource centre rang up all those who had the day off and asked them to come in. People ran round the room flapping bits of paper at each other. Office-based members of staff left the office and came to the control room to add to the sudden bustle of activity. I was left manning the 999 phones, wondering what on earth was going on and what I would get next.

At about 9.20 a.m. I took a call from a rather flustered-sounding policewoman, from Paddington Police Station.

'There's been an incident at Edgware Road underground station!' she said.

'An explosion?' I asked.

'How did you know?' she said, confused.

I explained that there had been explosions reported at umpteen other stations too, and we thought it was due to a power surge. At that point we didn't know how many explosions there had been, we only knew how many stations were affected (Liverpool Street, Aldgate, Aldgate East, King's Cross, Russell Square, and now Edgware Road and Paddington) so we thought the situation was even worse than it was. By now, we were starting to disbelieve the power surge theory. It simply didn't fit with the facts – why would a power surge affect stations on different lines, on opposite sides of the city, while intermediate stations were unaffected? Rumours and speculation abounded as calls came in from hospitals, the press and members of the public. Were there two separate bombs at Russell Square and King's Cross? Had the trains at Edgware Road collided? Had another bomb been found at Victoria? Had people been killed at Canary Wharf? Had a bus exploded near Euston?

We only knew the bus really had exploded when the first ambulance got there. All the 999 calls on the subject – all six of them – had been made from a building opposite (by this point the mobile networks were down), but the callers had been forced to hang up as they had been evacuated from the building. Only one had got as far as mentioning the exploded bus before they hung up. It was impossible to distinguish these calls from a cruel hoax or the count-less other rumours we'd received second-hand.

By 10 a.m. a state of organized pandemonium had crept in. Peo-ple in fluorescent coats were shouting things about death tolls and numbers of casualties. We took a steady stream of calls and just tried to deal with them one at a time. We refused to send ambu-lances to all but the most serious of calls, and even some of those declined our aid, saying that the bomb victims needed us more and that they'd make their own way to hospital. Even though they were in the middle of a heart attack.

Everyone was given just ten minutes out of the room to contact their relatives.

The first call I made was to my boyfriend, Alan, who works in Hammersmith. He'd gone through Edgware Road station just fif-teen minutes before the bomb went off.

He knew nothing about it.

'Thank goodness you're okay!' I exclaimed.

'Why on earth wouldn't I be?' he said, huffily. 'Why are you ringing me at work? You never ring me at work!'

'There's been ... things going on ... people dead ... explo-sions ... bombs!'

'Oh my God! Bombs?'

It didn't seem real until I'd said it. But then I looked at the scene before me. Waterloo Road was closed. Ambulance Control had been turned into Fort Knox with a battalion of ambulances block-ing the road, half the police force milling around on the steps and a big marquee full of important goings-on outside. I took in the scene before me: this was a real major incident – something people would remember for the rest of their lives – and there I was, right in the middle of it.

Things became eerily quiet in the control room around lunchtime. Manning was at full capacity but the call rate had actually gone down. There were no further explosions, all the ambulances were out dealing with casualties, and the general public had finally got the message and stopped calling. Mostly.

We all got to eat the free sandwiches which had mysteriously appeared from nowhere, and then it was decided we could start accepting calls again, although waiting times were horrific and London hospitals were only accepting emergency cases. GPs were sending those patients that couldn't wait for treatment to Welwyn Garden City, Watford, East Grinstead and the like.

I got a lift home in a Patient Transport ambulance as there were no tubes running. The driver got lost and kept driving in circles around Aldgate. There was no sign of what had happened there just ten hours ago, but I knew.

I'd seen the reports.

Fifty-two people had been killed today, and seven of them had been killed at Aldgate.

# The Essentials

# How the Ambulance System Works

I am an Emergency Medical Dispatcher. In other words, I am the person on the other end of the phone when you dial 999 for an ambulance. If you were to walk into the London Ambulance Service's control room – a dingy windowless pit housed in a 1970s monolith in Waterloo – and peer into the call-taking area, there I'd be, scribbling notes for this book on the back of a rejected annual leave slip. It surprises a lot of people to learn that call takers are the bottom of the Emergency Medical Dispatch hierarchy. Those who regularly work on the dispatch desks – that is, the people who actually send out the ambulances – are more experienced and better paid. This is mainly because they are making the decisions upon which people's lives depend. The call taker's job, on the other hand, is to follow protocol. The things we are supposed to find out and the instructions we give are all scripted. But there's one thing you can't write a script for, and that's finding those magic words that get through to callers and get them to do whatever is necessary to help the patient. That's where the real talent of an Emergency Medical Dispatcher lies. It's about staying calm and detached when chaos reigns on the other end of the phone, without giving the impression you don't care. It's about biting your tongue and staying professional when faced with timewasters. It's about treating all callers as equal yet different.

Although we're taught various techniques for calming people down and getting them to comply with instructions, you cannot teach someone to be a good call taker. Either you have it, or you don't – and a lot of people realize they don't.

EMDs have one of the highest turnover rates in the NHS.

I don't think anyone aspires to become an EMD. Have you ever asked a child what he wants to become when he grows up and heard him reply, 'I want to be the person who answers 999 calls'? I thought not. Most EMDs stumble across the job by accident. Some come from more physically demanding medical jobs which they are no longer able to perform due to ill health. Some think it will be good practice before a career with the police or fire brigade. Some are biding their time before becoming paramedics – the minimum age for paramedics in London is twenty-one. Some are attracted by the fact that the overtime and unsocial hours bonuses attract a fairly impressive wage for a job which requires no formal qualifications. For me, Emergency Medical Dispatch was a way out of the most boring admin job ever invented. I worked in the IT department of a London hospital, setting up logins for new staff members and explaining to computer illiterate midwives how to reboot their PC. The highlight of my day was being called out of my office to remove fluff from someone's mouse. I was bored and unfulfilled. I saw the nurses and doctors milling around the hospital, engrossed in their work, helping people, making a difference. But I couldn't become a nurse or a doctor. I was twenty-seven years old, I'd already been to university and got a (useless) degree; I simply didn't have the time or money for another bout of study.

Then my eyes wandered to A&E, to the ambulance bay outside where two jolly green-clad blokes were sipping tea outside a green-and-yellow-checked ambulance. I took in the blue lights, the stretcher, the oxygen cylinders ... I imagined the vehicle speeding to train crashes, to drowning children, house fires ... the excitement and exhilaration of saving lives without the need to go back to university. I could do that. Er, well, I could – except for one small detail. A paramedic needs to be able to drive the ambulance. And I cannot drive. A gruelling course of driving lessons a couple of years ago had, in fact, convinced me that I might never be able to drive.

My eyes fell to the next item on the Job Vacancies list. Emergency Medical Dispatchers. 999 bods! Now I could definitely do *that*! I wasn't quite sure what the job entailed other than answering 999 calls – and I wasn't sure how one answered a 999 call – but figuring that anything would be better than defluffing mice for the rest of my life, I sent off for an application pack.

A series of psychometric tests and a gruelling interview later, I was told my application was successful and sent away to Bow Headquarters with a bunch of other nervous newbies and taught items of varying interest, such as what you should do if the control room catches fire (nothing – you're not allowed to leave), how many ambulances get sent to initial reports of a plane crash (six) and the percentage of 999 calls that have a genuine medical need for an ambulance (forty). I was presented with an ill-fitting, starchy green uniform and packed off for a bit of on-the-job training with a more experienced EMD in the control room. Once I had reached a sufficient standard – that is, not likely to kill anyone, could recite CPR (cardiopulmonary resuscitation) instructions with eyes closed, could spell 'diarrhoea' without aid of medical dictionary – I was signed off and allowed to go it alone.

I'd been there nearly a year on 7 July 2005, the day of the London bombings. It was the day when I realized what I'd got myself into. How did it compare to setting up passwords and fixing mice? Do you even want me to answer that?

Despite the fact that I fell into this job – one that no one chooses and no one appreciates – I think it's the most amazing, enjoyable and rewarding job, and I wouldn't do any other. What other job gives you a window into the most intimate moments of strangers' lives – births, deaths, domestics, breakdowns and the occasional embarrassing sexual accident – and allows you to really make a difference? Where else can you just sit in front of a computer answering a telephone and still come home and say you saved a life at work today? Despite the fact that it sometimes has me tearing my hair out in frustration – or despairing at the state of the world – I wouldn't give it up for anything.

And with this book I hope to give you some insight into what it's like to do my job – and how you can help me to do it well.

# How Call Taking Works

Emergency Medical Dispatchers are the bête noire of emergency workers. We provide the sort of help people don't want. We ask people 'stupid questions' while their loved ones die in front of their eyes. We ask them to do impossible things. We don't know where they mean when they say 'outside Tesco's in East London'. We don't 'just send the ambulance'. We never get thank-you letters.

The problem is, it isn't like it is on TV. In soaps, characters often just call for an ambulance, bark an incomplete address and then hang up. And then – *nee naw nee naw nee naw* – the ambulance arrives, the crew bundle the patient into the back of the ambulance and save the day, and everyone lives happily ever after.

In real life, making a 999 call for an ambulance is considerably more like hard work – for both caller and call taker – and we EMDs are incredibly grateful to members of the public who make it easier. The problem callers, with a few exceptions, aren't malicious or stupid, they're just uneducated – and this isn't really their fault. If 'How to Call an Ambulance' was taught in schools or as part of first-aid courses, I'm sure people would be a lot better at it. If they realized that we ask questions and give instructions to help the caller, the patient and the ambulance crew, they wouldn't be so obstructive. But, of course, we only talk to people once they are faced with an emergency, and that's generally not when they're most receptive to a lecture about how the 999 system works.

But now I've got your attention, I'll explain it to you. And hopefully, when the time comes for you to make that call, you'll remember – we really are here to help you. We're here for you *as well as* the ambulance, not *instead of* the ambulance.

I'll talk you through what happens when you make a 999 call.

★

The first voice you'll hear is the Emergency Operator, who will say, 'Emergency – which service, please?'

The Emergency Operator works for the phone company, not for any of the emergency services, and will connect you to us as soon as you say 'ambulance'. (If you don't say which service you need, the operator will make an educated guess. If they have no idea at all, they will connect you to the police.)

The next voice you hear will be an Emergency Medical Dispatcher. (Not an 'operator'. EMDs hate being called 'operator' for much the same reason paramedics hate being called 'ambulance driver'. And besides, how can I be an operator when I can't even work a switchboard?)

The EMD will ask, 'What's the problem? Tell me exactly what happened.'

You should give a clear, concise answer. For instance: 'My grandmother has chest pain.' You should always mention 'priority symptoms' first if the patient has any of the following: chest pain, difficulty breathing, unconsciousness or uncontrolled bleeding. We prefer to hear symptoms rather than diagnoses – you might be quite sure that the person in front of you is having a heart attack, but we don't know what training you've had and what has led you to that belief.

There are some things you can say that are totally useless. One word that *sounds* quite informative, but actually isn't, is 'collapsed'. This is because people collapse for all kinds of reasons (heart attack, broken leg, shock at Leyton Orient winning a football match, etc.). Try to find out why the patient has collapsed.

But the absolutely least useful thing you can say is, 'It's a really serious emergency! Please come quickly! She's going to die!'

This is useless because the call taker has absolutely no control over the sending of the ambulance. All they can do is take the information you give and type it into the computer so the dispatch desk (which I will tell you about later) can see it and act on it. And believe me, no dispatch desk is going to be impressed by a diagnosis of *really serious emergency*. They've heard it all before. If you blather on like that, the call taker will be sitting with fingers poised

over the computer, ready to type, probably realizing from the tone
of your voice that it is indeed a really serious emergency, but pow-
erless to do anything until you say what the emergency is. A good
call taker will draw on their reserves of calming techniques to try
to find the right thing to say in order to get through to you, to
make you compose yourself and give the required information. A
skill you need for this job is the ability to work out just what that
is. Some callers want to hear you share their panic: 'Oh my God,
that's awful! Right, do as I say so we can help you!' Others need
you to sound calm, detached and in control: 'We deal with this all
the time. I'm just running through a few protocol questions here.'
And others need a concrete explanation: 'Tell me exactly what's
wrong so we can send the correct kind of help. We have different
kinds of ambulances for different things. While I'm talking to you,
my colleague upstairs is ringing the ambulance crew, so talking to
me won't delay help.'

Once a brief diagnosis is established, the call taker will ask you
for the address. Call takers have to play dumb at this point: if
you've called from a landline, they will already have it. But they
will insist you give the full address, including postcode area, so
that any mistakes will be yours and not theirs. If you clearly don't
know, they will secretly fill in the address while pretending to
remain oblivious and then send you to find out where you are.
This sometimes leads to ambulances turning up and surprising
people before they have even given an address.

You would be surprised at how many people shout 'Hurry up!'
before they have even given the address. Another line we hear surprisingly regularly is: 'Look, never mind the address, just send the
ambulance!' But until we input a precise address to the computer,
the call details won't appear on the screens on the dispatch desk, so
they won't even know the call exists.

Once we have an address and diagnosis, we have enough information to send an ambulance. But that's not the end of the call. The
call taker will ask you what a lot of callers think are a bunch of
stupid questions about whether the patient is conscious, breathing,
bleeding, clammy, pale, etc. The questions are all scripted – they're

from a protocol called AMPDS (Advanced Medical Priority Dispatch System) which was developed in America and is used throughout the world. Which questions you are asked depends on what you initially said was wrong with the patient. Because they're scripted, some of the questions sound a bit strange – for instance, if you dislocate your shoulder, you will be asked if it is bleeding, because that question is always asked for traumatic injuries.

Some callers query the usefulness of the questions or, worse still, refuse to answer. They say it's wasting time – which is ridiculous, because it generally takes far less time to answer the questions than to get into a debate about how useful they are. There are three important reasons for asking these questions:

1. To convey information to the ambulance crew, so they know exactly where to start when they arrive and don't have to waste their time asking questions.
2. To allow the computer to triage the call, so that ambulances are sent to the most important calls first (I'll explain more about call categories later).
3. To help the call taker assess what you need to do while waiting for the ambulance and whether you need to be given any instructions.

Once you've answered the questions, you can give the call taker any other information that you think is relevant. We need to know, for example, if the patient weighs forty stone or if you live on the twentieth floor of a building with a broken lift. (Let's hope those two don't occur in combination.) We don't need to know about the patient's medical history unless it's something really unusual or relevant to the current problem. That sort of information is useful to the ambulance crew and the doctors, but not to us. It's funny, but while some callers refuse to answer any questions, others insist on telling you every single irrelevant detail they can muster, to the point where they don't hear the ambulance arriving because they are too engrossed in the phone call.

★

After you've answered all the questions, the call taker will give you instructions on what to do next. For most calls, where the patient is stable and nothing more can be done until the ambulance arrives, the instructions go as follows.

Reassure her help is being arranged, watch her closely, get her medication and doctor's details ready, turn the lights on, open the door, send someone to meet the ambulance and if her condition worsens in any way, call us back immediately for further instructions!

It's a sentence I must have read out hundreds of thousands of times. It's not meant to be all one sentence but my tongue goes into autopilot.

On calls where the patient's condition is deteriorating, the EMD will stay on the line and give first-aid instructions until the ambulance arrives. EMDs can tell you how to do CPR, how to maintain the airway of an unconscious patient, what to do when someone is fitting, how to control bleeding, what to do if someone is choking and how to deliver a baby. We even have a protocol for what to do if someone is in a sinking vehicle. Strangely enough, I've never used it.

Frustratingly, while this is the part of the call where the EMD can make the most difference, it is also the part where we are met with the most opposition. A sizeable proportion of callers do not want to 'do something'. They want *us* to turn up and do something. They want it to be like it is in Soapland – where they put the phone down and the ambulance crew come running in. They think that if they start doing something themselves, you'll tell them, 'See, you're doing fine. No need for an ambulance, then.' They think that because they're not trained, they'll make things worse, even though in a lot of cases the patient is *definitely* going to die if they don't do anything – they can't possibly make it worse. They think that putting the phone down is going to make you abandon the idea of giving these ridiculous instructions and instead do what you should have been doing all along – getting an ambulance there.

It won't – that's not our job. Someone else is busy upstairs doing that.

If the caller hangs up, we just ring them back. If we're not too busy banging our heads against the desk in frustration, that is.

For some reason, a lot of people are convinced that you can't possibly be organizing help and giving instructions at the same time. This is not helped by the fact that we are under strict instructions not to mention one particular 'Forbidden Phrase'. That phrase is: 'The ambulance is on its way.' We can't say this, even when we know full well the ambulance *is* on its way, because, according to Management, it increases expectations that an ambulance will be sent, whereas in fact they might get a visit from an adviser, an Emergency Care Practitioner in a car, or even a helicopter turning up. A lot of the time, though, callers are so set in their expectations that nothing we say will change them, and sometimes the Forbidden Phrase is exactly what they need to hear. So, very occasionally, I say it.

Another problem is that some people seem to think there is only one person working for the Ambulance Service. Because they can't hear anyone activating an ambulance, they assume one is not being sent. It doesn't seem to occur to them that it is all done silently, by computer, even though pretty much everything in the world can be done by computer these days. Some people even think you are going to jump in the ambulance at the end of the call and come round yourself. I sometimes think that I should do something to convince the callers that help really is coming – pretend to put them on hold while I summon an ambulance, even imitate a nee naw siren fading off into the distance – just to convince them that an Emergency Medical Dispatcher's help really is help and not a fob-off.

Of course, there are callers who do get it right, and they are like a breath of fresh air. It's so refreshing when someone just answers your questions with a simple yes or no and doesn't try to hurry you along. It's unbelievably rewarding when you hear the panic subside in someone's voice and they do their best to follow your instructions. It's even better when they remember to thank you at the end of the call. Those calls where everything goes right make all the stressful ones worthwhile.

# Call Categories and Appropriate Responses

When the call taker has entered all of the caller's answers to the AMPDS questions into the computer, the computer will give the call a category based on the answers. There are three categories of call, and the way in which the Ambulance Service handle each call category is different.

## *Red Calls*

These are also referred to as category A (Cat A) and are classified as 'immediately life-threatening'. According to government targets, we have eight minutes to reach them. Examples of red calls are heart attacks, asthma attacks, anaphylactic shock (a severe type of allergic reaction), breech births, cardiac arrests, suspected meningitis and head injuries with reduced consciousness. A rule of thumb is that *any* call where the patient is having difficulty breathing, chest pain or is losing consciousness will be a red call. Some frequent callers have cottoned on to this and say one of these things is happening just to make the ambulance come faster. I just hope they think of the effect this might have on a caller with a genuine emergency who has to wait longer as a result.

The dispatch desk's response to a red call is simple: get there as quickly as possible. We send the nearest available ambulance, which might mean diverting one that was on its way to a lower priority call if necessary. If there is no ambulance available, we pull out all the stops to find one, which usually entails the radio operator making what is known as a GB (general broadcast) – basically 'advertising' the call on the radio in the hope that an ambulance crew finishing off their paperwork or having a quick break will tell us they are able to run on it.

We don't just send ambulances, either – FRUs (fast/first response units, otherwise known as ambulance cars) are sent to the most urgent calls because they get there faster. FRUs are staffed by one paramedic or an emergency medical technician (EMT). Once the ambulance arrives, they finish up and become available for the next call. Because they don't go to hospital, they have a much quicker turnaround. FRUs are run by their own desk. The FRU desk also has responders on motorcycles and pushbikes (they have a mini version of an ambulance kit in a basket on the back of their bike). Bike ambulances are particularly useful in the heart of London, shopping centres and Heathrow airport, where there are either no roads at all for regular ambulances to get down, or narrow, busy roads where regular ambulances can be delayed for a long time in traffic.

Serious trauma calls – that is, nasty road traffic accidents, stabbings, shootings, amputations, hangings, that sort of thing – may also get the Helicopter Emergency Medical Service (HEMS). It takes off from the Royal London Hospital in Whitechapel and usually has a doctor, a paramedic and two pilots on board. They do amazing things such as cutting people open and performing lifesaving surgery at the roadside. HEMS, incidentally, is a charity and relies on donations from the public to keep doing its very important work. It costs £1,000 every time HEMS is dispatched to a call, but it really is worth it – in cases of serious trauma, getting the patient to the hospital can kill them. HEMS effectively brings the hospital to them. There are no EMDs directly involved with HEMS, but they have their own desk within our control room, staffed by paramedics, so they communicate with us better.

## Amber Calls

Also known as category B (Cat B), these are calls that are 'serious but not *immediately* life-threatening'. These include minor strokes, diabetic hypos, broken bones, uncontrollable bleeding, some road traffic accidents, people threatening suicide, and overdoses. We treat amber calls much the same as we treat red calls, except it isn't quite such a national emergency if we don't get to them straight away. The FRU desk doesn't have to send FRUs to amber calls; they decide on an individual basis after looking at the diagnosis and how quickly an ambulance will be able to get there. The government target for this type of call is nineteen minutes.

## Green Calls

Finally, we have green calls – category C (Cat C) – which are defined as 'neither serious nor life-threatening'. There are no government targets determining how quickly we reach them. A lot of green calls are misuse of the service, but a lot – for instance, elderly people lying on the floor with a hip injury – are appropriate, and I sometimes wish an ambulance could be sent to them before some of the red and amber calls! Examples of green calls are sprained ankles, flu, paper cuts on fingers, diarrhoea and vomiting (the ailment 90 per cent of call takers cannot spell), an elderly person who has fallen and has no injuries but can't get up, and doctors' calls for someone (usually elderly) who needs admitting to hospital, for example for a chest infection, whose condition is stable but who can't get to hospital without an ambulance.

Green calls are usually dealt with by UOC (Urgent Operations Centre), another smaller control room in the same building which deals with the lower priority calls. The first people to look at the call will be CTA (Clinical Telephone Advice).

CTA are paramedics who ring back the caller and advise them on what to do (home care advice, seeing their GP, making their own way to hospital, etc.). If CTA decide the call does need an ambulance (or if the caller insists on having one anyway – we can't say no) the call is passed on to UOC, who can send a 'Green Truck'.

A Green Truck looks like a normal ambulance from the outside, but has less equipment on board, and the technicians who run it have less training and skills than normal technicians and paramedics. A Green Truck therefore costs the service less to run, and an advantage of having them is that the deserving green calls – old people on the floor, and the like – do not have to wait until there are no red/amber calls outstanding before they get an ambulance, because Green Trucks can't deal with those anyway.

If there are no Green Trucks available, the call gets passed back down to us in the main control room, and we send an emergency ambulance as soon as we have one available. Needless to say, if the diagnosis is 'paper cut on finger' and the only reason we have to send an ambulance is because CTA couldn't talk the patient out of having an ambulance (and all the Green Trucks are busy), we get a bit annoyed.

So that's how it all works.

Now I'm going to share with you two years of being on the other end of the 999 call – my hopes, my fears, my firsts. I hope by the end of it you'll know just what it's like to be an Emergency Medical Dispatcher. And why I'd never do anything else.

2005

# My First BBA

Five hundred million billion calls to suspect packages in the last week. I am sick of them. Fortunately, I was distracted today by fulfilling something which has been an ambition of mine since my first day at Ambulance Control. I delivered my first baby!

The location, weirdly enough, was the toilets of the Leek and Winkle pub in Romford. I actually went to this pub not so long ago and it has the most amazing toilets with wall-length mirrors, spotlighting and plush couches. The poor mother-to-be had been out shopping – not the most sensible thing to do when you are nine months pregnant, I must say – and had suddenly gone into labour. She'd headed for the nearest pub to seek help. A member of staff had called 999 straight away, but as the patient had rushed to the toilet, no one realized how close she was to giving birth and the call was classified as green, meaning we'd not sent anyone yet. All the ambulances were probably out dealing with bloomin' suspect package calls instead.

After going back to check on the mother, the barmaid realized that the baby was going to make an entrance sooner rather than later. She called 999 again and it was me who answered. After getting enough details to find her original call, I went through the questions again to see if the call needed upgrading. The signs all pointed towards 'delivery imminent' but I wasn't getting excited. I'd heard this all before. A lot of people insist the mother is having contractions less than a minute apart when really she is walking around with her tights on and won't deliver until sometime next week.

Well, that wasn't the case here. I found this out when I asked the barmaid to look between the mother's legs. (An unenviable task!)

'I can see the head!' she exclaimed.

It was all systems go from that point. I pulled up the maternity card on the computer and rattled off the instructions.

**Me: AS THE BABY'S HEAD DELIVERS, GENTLY PLACE THE PALM OF YOUR HAND AGAINST THE VAGINA TO PREVENT IT DELIVERING TOO QUICKLY.**

**Barmaid: OKAY ... IT'S COMING OUT! WHAT NEXT?**

**Me: SUPPORT THE BABY'S HEAD AND SHOULDERS AS IT DELIVERS. REMEMBER, THE BABY WILL BE SLIPPERY – DON'T DROP IT!**

**Baby: WAAAAAAAAAAAH!!!!**

Fortunately, it was a straightforward birth – head first, cord not around neck, crying straight away, and all that needed to be done was to wrap the baby in a towel and give her to her shell-shocked mother. I was amazed at how little time it took between the head appearing and the rest of the baby being out.

The ambulance crew entered seconds after the birth, right on cue, so I didn't have to faff around with the cord and afterbirth, which is a good thing. One step at a time!

My first BBA (born before arrival) is an important milestone for me. I was beginning to wonder what was going on because I have managed to work here for a whole year without having one. One of the girls who started at the same time as me has already had six! My other milestones were my first cardiac arrest (which I had in my first week), my first cardiac arrest in a non-elderly person (which was a terminally ill eight-year-old – the way the parents seemed resigned to his death broke my heart), my first stabbing (utter chaos), my first rude person (an elderly man who was waiting for an ambulance to take him to a routine hospital appointment and didn't understand that emergencies come first). I'm still waiting for an embarrassing sexual accident, a suicide and a drowning! Not that I'm going to enjoy any of these things, of course – but I know they are coming and I know I need to get them over with. I want to know that I am able to cope with *anything*.

The most horrible milestone that I haven't completed yet is my first cot death call, and I know it'll happen soon. I think that's the call that everyone dreads more than anything.

# Embarrassing Sexual Accidents I

## 18 July 2005

Since delivering my first baby, my Call-taking Ambition has moved on to the next item on the list: the Embarrassing Sexual Accident. This was fulfilled late on Saturday night, when I received a call from a rather shamefaced, tearful gentleman in an embarrassing predicament. The man's girlfriend had 'got a bit carried away' with a vibrator and now the offending sex aid was lodged deep inside his anal passage. Understandably, he was extremely ashamed of the mess he had got himself into. I tried to convince him that we see this kind of thing every day and in no way would the A&E staff, ambulance crew and entire population of Ambulance Control be sniggering about this until the end of the shift. I wish this were true, but in fact such incidents aren't that common – at least, from an ambulance point of view. (I suspect the majority of those thus afflicted go to A&E by taxi, thus reducing the number of people they have to explain the problem to.) His was, in fact, the first lost vibrator I have encountered so far (a few months ago, the person next to me took a call about a hairspray can stuck in a vagina, but that is as close as I've got), but I didn't think it would be prudent to share this fact with him, nor exclaim: 'All the way up! That's kind of impressive!'

Neither did I ask the question which was on everyone's lips for the rest of the night, which was: 'Is the vibrator still switched on?'

Anyway, the poor man told me that the embarrassment was too much, that he couldn't face waking up his small children and being subjected to an inquisition from them (the perpetrating girlfriend had fled the premises, leaving him right in the lurch) and that he would try to remove it himself (I didn't enquire how). I suggested that he ring NHS Direct for advice. I don't suppose they were able to help – but they are always referring calls to us, so I thought I'd refer someone back to them for a change.

About an hour later, the man rang back and came through to Snowy, sitting a few desks down from me. He had conceded defeat and the call priority had now gone up from a green 'object stuck' to a red 'dangerous haemorrhage' due to rectal bleeding. An ambulance was dispatched (I bet the dispatch desk deliberately chose an all-female crew) but the man remained very concerned about his children. He didn't want to bring them with him, nor place them in the care of his girlfriend or anyone else. At this point he let slip to Snowy that his wife was away, and the penny dropped that his reluctance to agree to medical help was not just embarrassment at having the cast of Casualty poke around his passageways but also the fact that when his wife returned, he was going to have some serious explaining to do as to who was inserting a vibrator into his rectum while she was on holiday and their two small children were asleep in the next room …

He could always give it the old 'I slipped and fell on a cucumber' line, I suppose.

# Fame at Last – or Not

The baby I helped deliver in the Leek and Winkle toilets last week has been featured in the *Romford Gazette*! There is a picture of her and the barmaid. They have called her Annabel, thus shattering my hopes of having a baby I helped deliver named after me. In fact, my contribution has not been mentioned at all.

Samantha, the barmaid, is quoted as saying: 'I rang for an ambulance, but they told me they were very busy and couldn't get an ambulance there for half an hour, so I hung up and took charge of the situation myself.'

I bet that's not what she said at all, but 'Heroic Barmaid Saves Day' makes a better story than 'Emergency Medical Dispatcher Does Job Properly'. Anyway, I don't care. I know what really happened – and besides, anyone who is anybody has been misquoted by the press at some point.

# Introducing Brenda

The average person will only have to call 999 for an ambulance once in their lifetime. There are some people, however, who feel compelled to dial us on an almost daily basis – so much so that we get to remember their names and addresses and instantly recognize them when their details flash up on our screens. Just in case the call taker is new or suffering from amnesia, our computer system has a way of flagging these addresses so that when we receive a call, we can read a little paragraph about the patient which will alert us as to what to expect.

One such caller is Brenda Kramer. Her paragraph reads as follows.

Brenda Kramer. Forty-two years old. Alcoholic, timewaster, regular caller. Has been abusive towards crews in past. Send police.

Today when Brenda called, she sounded in a bad way. Her speech was slurred, she was confused and stuttering.

'What's the problem, Brenda?' I asked. 'Tell me exactly what's happened.'

In stilted speech Brenda slowly explained. She'd suddenly got a terrible headache, she was numb down one side, she was dizzy and her memory was shot to pieces. She felt terrible and she didn't know why. She couldn't even walk, she thought we'd have to kick the door down.

All the signs of a stroke, I thought: poor Brenda really was sick this time. I was relieved to see the call came out as a red call and an ambulance was sent straight away. Her condition sounded really serious.

An hour later I checked back on the call to see how Brenda was doing. What I saw surprised me. There, against 'outcome', the crew had recorded: 'Declined aid against advice.' But that couldn't be right! She had sounded desperate for help, and surely the crew wouldn't just leave her if she was having a stroke.

I ran up to the dispatch desk to ask them about the call.

'Oh dear, don't tell me you haven't encountered Brenda before?' smiled Jenny, the allocator (allocators are the most senior people on the dispatch desk). 'She does tend to be very convincing the first few times you encounter her. She's obviously read a medical encyclopedia, because every time she rings she reels off the symptoms of a serious ailment like a heart attack or stroke – but when the crew examine her, there's never anything wrong. I think she just calls us because she is bored. She never, ever goes to hospital.'

I am sad to say that I was completely taken in. Next time I will save my sympathy for someone who really deserves it.

# Embarrassing Sexual Accidents II

7 August 2005

The man with the vibrator stuck up his bottom should count himself lucky. Some sexual accidents are beyond embarrassing. At 11 a.m. this morning I received a call from a young girl living in a town on the outskirts of London. She spoke with a timid, mousy, on-the-verge-of-tears voice, and explained that there was something wrong with her 21-year-old boyfriend. He'd been fine one minute, the next his body had gone into spasm, he was stiff as a board, turning blue and making a choking noise. My initial thought was that the boyfriend was having some kind of fit, although the symptoms weren't that of an epileptic fit (or anything else I'd ever heard of) – his body was rigid, rather than jerking. I categorized the call using the unconsciousness protocol and it came out as a red. The boyfriend obviously wasn't breathing very well, but I wasn't terribly worried about this at first because of the fit-like symptoms – people who are fitting tend not to breathe properly, but they recover without any intervention.

While I was waiting for the spasms to stop, I asked the mousy girl for some background information. She told me that they'd been out last night, they had been drinking but not taking drugs, and had been doing what couples usually do on a Sunday morning if they're too hung-over to get out of bed, when the incident occurred. (I don't mean that they were ordering pizza on their laptop, I mean they were having sexual intercourse.)

Then the girl informed me that the boyfriend had stopped spasming and was now lying still, so I told her to get him into the ready-for-CPR position, expecting that the boyfriend would now start to recover. Instead she informed me that he was now breathing very faintly and making a soft gurgling sound, and that his breathing was definitely getting worse. At this point I began to suspect that the gurgling and choking noises described throughout the call had not been harmless fitting-related sounds but in fact the ominous 'death rattle' – the horrible sound someone makes when their last breath escapes from their lungs as they die. (Unfortunately, the patient wasn't close enough to the phone for me to hear for myself.) I asked her to check whether he was breathing, and she was all over the place – 'Yes, I think so, but I'm not sure . . . I think he's stopping . . . I can't tell! I can feel some warmth coming out!' I was in two minds about whether to start CPR (if the patient is breathing, it's really not a good thing to be doing to them) and sent her back to check again. Then there were sirens, a buzz at the door, footsteps and talking. The girl was heard to squeak, 'He's not breathing! He's not breathing!' and then I got a tap on the shoulder to confirm that the buzz at the door had been the FRU and that I could hang up now. I turned round to find half of Ambulance Control peering over my shoulder.

As soon as I had my break, I went up to the dispatch desk to see if they'd heard any more. Apparently the boyfriend had been in cardiac arrest when the crew arrived, but they had managed to zap him with a defibrillator and get his heart beating again. He was still not breathing by himself. He was rushed into hospital in this state, with a normal pulse but very low blood pressure.

A few hours later I got a call from the allocator. The boyfriend had died in hospital. Not only that, but the police were treating the death as suspicious. I don't know why they thought it was suspicious – perhaps just by virtue of the fact that 21-year-old men do not usually drop dead for no good reason. Speculation, as you can imagine, was rife for the rest of the afternoon as to what had caused this untimely demise.

It's funny after you get a call like this. You're allowed to take a break if you're feeling upset by it, but I find the best thing for me is just to plough on and not dwell on events. The next call is always guaranteed to be someone ranting and raving because they called an ambulance for their stomach ache ten minutes ago, so why isn't it here yet? It is always difficult not to tell them to bog off and give them a lecture about dying people and what ambulances are really for. While your life is going on as normal, you have been listening in on the moment that will change the life of someone just like you for ever. That morning the girl and her boyfriend were a normal couple – like me and my boyfriend, Alan – and now he is in a fridge somewhere and she is being investigated by the police.

I got home and Alan was feeling a bit amorous, but I told him I had a headache. You can't be too careful.

# A Good Day

13 August 2005

It was getting to the last hour in the shift from hell and I answered the phone in the usual way to hear a very small voice on the other end of the line.

Her: HELLO ... I'M SORRY TO BOTHER YOU, AMBULANCE SERVICE, BUT I CAN'T GET HOLD OF MY GP ... AND I THINK I NEED SOMEONE TO CHECK ME OVER TO SEE IF I'M ALRIGHT.

Me: (SLIGHTLY CONFUSED.) WELL, WHAT'S WRONG? ARE YOU ILL? IN PAIN? HAD AN ACCIDENT?

Her: NO ... NO ... I HAVE A MENTAL HEALTH PROBLEM.

Me: (PENNY DROPS.) AH! WELL, WHAT SEEMS TO BE THE PROBLEM? ARE YOU DEPRESSED? SUICIDAL? PARANOID? DO YOU HAVE A RADIO IN YOUR HEAD CONTROLLED BY FIDEL CASTRO?* WE COULD SEND YOU AN AMBULANCE TO CHECK YOU OVER, IF YOU LIKE?

Her: NO ... NO ... I DON'T WANT AN AMBULANCE ... ER ...

Me: HOW ABOUT CALLING THE EMERGENCY DOCTOR, THEN?

Her: WELL, ACTUALLY ... IT'S NOT AN EMERGENCY ... I JUST WANTED TO TALK TO SOMEONE ...

Me: HOW ABOUT THE SAMARITANS, THEN? THEY'RE REALLY GOOD TO TALK TO AND CAN HELP YOU IF YOU'RE FEELING SAD OR LONELY.

Her: UM, NO ... YOU SEE, I'M NOT ... I ACTUALLY HAD A REALLY GOOD DAY (STARTS TO CRY) AND ... I JUST WANTED TO TELL SOMEONE ... I DON'T VERY OFTEN HAVE GOOD DAYS, YOU SEE ... I JUST WANTED SOMEONE TO TELL ME I'M GOING TO BE ALRIGHT ...

* I didn't actually say that about Fidel Castro. I am using a bit of poetic licence here. I do that sometimes.

# An Invitation

Oh my God! I got home at 7.30 a.m. after a particularly gruelling night shift to find an invitation on my doormat to an 'Emergency Services Reception' at 10 Downing Street. It seems they've picked me as I took the first call on 7 July – that insignificant-seeming request for an ambulance on standby from the fire brigade! I'm going to meet Tony Blair! I am in shock! And the dress code says 'lounge suit'. I don't even know what a lounge suit is.

# Cot Death

Today I had my first cot death.

Since I've been at Ambulance Control, this is the call I've been dreading. Cot deaths tend to come in at the very beginning of a day shift or the very end of a night shift – around 7 a.m. – because this is the time the baby's mother or father wakes up (perhaps having had a short lie-in because for once the baby isn't crying) and finds them dead in their cot. Around this time of day the phone lines are quiet because most of the world is asleep, and those who do call in have just woken up and want to be spoken to in a quiet voice. The sound of the call taker receiving the cot death will ring out above those sleepy whispers, and every time it's happened I've thanked the gods of ambulances that that call didn't come through to me and prayed that my next call will be a nice old lady who's fallen out of bed. Up until now every call I've had about a patient who isn't breathing ('suspended' we call it) has been either an old person or someone who has been involved in a road traffic accident. Of course, I don't place more value on a child's life than on anyone else's, but there is a certain horror in the death of a child, which isn't there when an eighty-year-old passes away. As soon as you become aware of death, you realize that one day you're going to have to face the death of your parents and grandparents, but no one bargains that they are going to face the death of the child – especially with no prior warning, before the child has even had a chance to live.

One day it had to be me who got the call. It happened just after 7 a.m., at the beginning of my first shift of the week. Actually, it wasn't nearly as bad as I had been expecting (for me, that is – it was as bad as you could get for the baby and his family). The baby's mother wasn't exactly *calm*, but she did still have her wits about her and figured that answering the questions and doing as she was told would get her further than screaming 'Ambulance, ambulance, ambulance!' as a lot of callers do. Then a neighbour arrived on the scene, so we were able to coordinate CPR and meeting the ambulance with military precision. The ambulance in fact took less than five minutes to arrive (although five minutes seems like five hours at times like these) and the situation did not get out of hand. There was no hysteria, no mention of death, all efforts were concentrated on doing everything for the child.

I went up to the dispatch desk to ask what had happened next – all they could tell me was that the baby had been rushed into hospital with the paramedics still trying to resuscitate him. That doesn't mean much, though, as they tend to take any non-breathing baby to hospital, even if it's been dead for a week, just in case. When I am in cynical mode, I think this is just to avoid any chance of being sued, but I suppose it must be a comfort to the baby's parents to know absolutely everything was done and that we didn't give up easily.

I volunteered myself to take calls from doctors making routine ambulance bookings for the next few hours – that call was quite enough drama for one day.

Just as I was packing up to go home, one of the allocators came down and told me that the baby didn't survive. This was as I suspected. She said there was nothing I (or anyone else, for that matter) could have done and that the baby had probably been dead hours by the time he was found. Sometimes a call will play on my mind at the end of the day and I will go home and keep thinking about it until I go to bed. It's only when I go back to work and take some more calls that I'm able to wipe it out. This wasn't one of them. I am beginning to realize that it is not the content of the call that can be disturbing, but the feeling that I could have done more, or that it was something I did that meant the patient didn't survive. Even if it's the caller's behaviour that caused the problem, it is still my job to calm them down and get them to do the best

thing for the patient. That wasn't the case in this call. I did everything right, the baby's mother did everything right, the neighbour did everything right, the ambulance turned up well ahead of
schedule, and no doubt the crew and hospital staff also did everything right.

And yet a one-month-old baby still died.

# I Told Him Not to Do it

Nine minutes to seven, and one last call before going home. It couldn't get any worse after starting the day with a cot death, could it? But what happened to these parents was worse – at least, to listen to. The mother made the initial call, she was crying too much to be understood. Fortunately, she was ringing from her landline, so I managed to decipher the address. When she sobbed, 'My son ... not breathing,' I had visions of another cot death, but then I asked the age.

'Fourteen,' she wailed.

I was about to instruct her on CPR, but suddenly she had a brainwave and shouted, almost unintelligibly, 'I'm a first-aider! I'm going to do resuscitation,' and then she dropped the phone and ran off to do it.

In the background I heard, faintly at first, shouting and banging. I thought there was a fight going on and that this was how the son came to be in such a predicament, but as the source of the noise approached the phone I realized this was the patient's father, who was utterly, utterly hysterical and smashing things. The man grabbed the phone and shouted the address down it, again and again. He didn't let me get a word in edgeways and it was as if he couldn't hear what I was saying to him at all. I eventually got his attention by bellowing in a very loud voice, which could probably be heard in the ambulance station below. It's never nice to have to bellow at people whose relatives are seriously ill, but sometimes you have to be cruel to be kind – increased volume is the only way to get their attention, and getting their attention might just achieve that piece of communication that saves the patient's life. While having his attention, I asked what had happened. It was very hard to understand what he was saying at first. Then I realized he was describing the appearance of his son. Face purple, eyes wide, unblinking, popping out of his head, bleeding from the mouth, stiff, cold, dead. I had to (inwardly) admit, it didn't sound as if there was much chance.

It felt like the longest call of my life. The worst time to call for an ambulance is 18.51, because many of the crews are on changeover at that time. It only adds a couple of minutes to the response time, but when you are trying to comfort the hysterical parents of a dead teenager, two minutes is a very long time.

The man continued howling and wailing and repeating himself and not making much sense. I gathered that he'd just come home and found his son like that, earlier the son had gone to do [something] and his father had told him not to do [whatever it was]. Whatever the patient had been doing was lost in the midst of hysterics, but he told him not to do it, he told him not to. He was my only son, he was my life, he is dead [crunch, bang], I told him not to do it.

The ambulance arrived at 19.01. It was the longest ten-minute phone call of my entire career.

# Death by Milkshake

I couldn't sleep last night thinking about the fourteen-year-old boy who'd died. Weirdly, it affected me far more than the cot death. Perhaps it was the way that sentence hung in the air: 'I told him not to do it.' What did he tell him not to do? I spoke to the ambulance crew who'd attended, and I told them what I'd heard on the phone.

'The scene was exactly as you described it,' said Steve, the paramedic. 'I've never witnessed such grief and it was really heartbreaking. The lad was clearly beyond all help when we got there but we gave it our best shot anyway – just so the parents would know we did everything we could. From what I could tell, he'd aspirated on a milkshake – that means it "went down the wrong way", into his lungs, and stopped him breathing. He basically choked to death.'

'That's terrible,' I said. 'I can't believe it was something so simple. Oh, one more thing. His dad kept saying on the phone, "I told him not to do it." What did he tell him not to do?'

'Drugs,' said Steve. 'There was some cannabis by his bed – I'm guessing he was having a spliff, got the munchies, went for one of those thick shakes but was so drowsy he didn't drink it properly, and that's how he died. His father must have thought it was the drugs that killed him, but really it was the milkshake.'

'Death by milkshake,' I said solemnly. 'What a waste.'

And we were both silent.

# Preparing for Number Ten

I went out yesterday and spent £100 on a new suit, consisting of a shiny red pencil skirt and matching jacket with a contrasting lacy black shirt, ready for my trip to Number Ten tomorrow. When I got home, I tried it on and asked Alan for his opinion. He laughed his head off and said I looked like I was going to a job interview. My mother came round later and assured me that it was very nice and well worth an entire day's wages.

Today I had a call from Management telling me that I was to be wearing dress uniform (a yucky green blazer and A-line skirt, not unlike my school uniform) and that I had to go in today – on my day off – to collect it! They could have told me this before I shelled out for the new suit. So I went into work and, of course, the person in charge had no idea what I was talking about. Dress uniform what? Number Ten where? I was just about to shuffle off home when I bumped into an equally confused-looking ambulance crew, who were also on the hunt for dress uniforms. Apparently they had been the first crew on the scene at Aldgate. They looked very impressed when I told them that I took 'The First Call'. I didn't tell them how boring that first call actually was. We eventually found the Dress Uniforms Department in an office five minutes' walk from the control room. They had just given out the last one in my size, so I had to go one bigger. It was a trifle baggy and my skirt almost reached the floor. I have been instructed to wear beige tights with it. Yuck.

# A Visit to Number Ten

8 September 2005

The coach to Downing Street left half an hour late because we were waiting for Peter Bradley, Chief of the Ambulance Service, otherwise known as The Boss. I said we should have issued him with a Late Report, since we get one if we are so much as three minutes late for work. Everyone sat looking very prim and nervous, twiddling their fingers in anticipation of meeting the Prime Minister and talking about anything except bombs. On arrival we were all scanned and X-rayed, mobile phones were confiscated, and we trooped through that infamous black door into Number Ten. As everyone says, it is much bigger on the inside than it appears on the outside, and the state rooms are as grand as you'd expect them to be, with great big sparkly chandeliers and antique chairs everywhere. One of the ambulance crews joked about stealing them and selling them on eBay. At least, I think they were joking.

Once inside, we were presented with an unlimited supply of white/red wine, orange juice or fizzy mineral water. As soon as you got halfway through your glass, a waiter appeared to top it up. Canapés also kept appearing, with stuff such as smoked salmon and duck in them. Some of the ambulance crews might have become rather tipsy, and everyone started to relax and talk to each other. Really, it was just like being at a party in a very posh house, where you didn't know anyone, and you had to wear your uniform. We discovered that one ambulance crew had been invited from each bombing, plus two people from Ambulance Control (me and someone from Management who was in charge of the control room that day) and some members of Senior Management with multiple pips on their shoulders. (I had no idea who they were or what they did.) I was surprised that it was just the two of us from Control – there were people working shifts that day who had done far more than I had – but I was glad they had invited someone, as Control's contribution often gets forgotten. And after all, if it wasn't for us, no one would ever get an ambulance!

I did feel like a bit of a fraud when we went round discussing what we'd done that day – 'I did CPR on a woman whose legs had been blown off and saved her life'; 'I treated a woman whose eye had been blown out of its socket and was hanging down to her chin'; 'Oh, I took a few phone calls' – especially as The First Call had been so insignificant, but I beefed it all up and made it sound more impressive and everyone was very nice and no one told me that I was rubbish and shouldn't be there or anything.

Other people in attendance included people from the fire brigade and the police, lots of staff from London Underground and London Buses, including the driver of the bus that blew up and the driver of the bus that took all the walking wounded from Aldgate to the Royal London Hospital. There were A&E nurses and doctors, surgeons who operated on the bomb victims, Dr Gareth Davies, who is in charge of HEMS, forensics people, the Salvation Army and lots of politicians. Apparently Charles Clarke was there but I didn't know what he looked like. A very drunk man from the Home Office came and talked to us about twenty-four-hour alcohol licensing and the effect it would have on the Ambulance Service. One of the paramedics said, 'I bet you're looking forward to it.'

At about 8 p.m. Tony Blair got up on a podium and made a speech about how wonderful we are. He doesn't look as good in real life as he does in his publicity photos. His speech went on a bit and had a lot of stuff I didn't see the point of, such as a discussion of the paintings in the state rooms. Maybe he'd been at the free wine too.

After this the ambulance crew from Aldgate (who'd helped me find the dress uniforms) and I decided we were going to ambush Mr Blair and make him speak to us. This was difficult as lots of pushy people kept getting in front of us, but eventually we managed to sidle in front of him. He shook all our hands, and then we had the following conversation.

**Mr Blair:** SO, YOU'RE FROM THE AMBULANCE SERVICE?

**Us:** (GORMLESS NODS ALL ROUND.)

**Mr Blair:** YOU MUST HAVE SEEN SOME HORRIBLE THINGS THAT DAY.

**Us:** (MORE GORMLESS NODS.)

**Mr Blair:** BUT THEN, I SUPPOSE YOU SEE A LOT OF HORRIBLE THINGS.

**Us:** (EVEN MORE GORMLESS NODS.)

**Random Fireman:** (BUTTING IN.) MR BLAIR! I WANT TO RAISE SOME ISSUES WITH YOU ABOUT THE MEMORIAL SERVICE AT ST PAUL'S ... I THOUGHT IT WAS DISGUSTING THAT THE FIRE BRIGADE WEREN'T MENTIONED ... BLAH BLAH ... APPALLING ... BLAH ...

And then Mr Blair was spirited away to talk about this perceived oversight, and that was that. Still, at least I got to tell my mother I'd met him!

On the coach back everyone was in high spirits and sitting backwards on the seats singing 'Ten Green Bottles'. It was just like a school trip, but with no teachers to keep order. The nice ambulance crew from Shoreditch took me to the pub and bought me drinks. There were some other ambulance crews there and I got talking to Steve, the paramedic who'd dealt with the 'death by milkshake' call. He offered to let me come out with him for a shift on his ambulance so I can see the calls they go to first hand! I am really excited about this – I often wonder what the ambulance crews actually get up to once we've sent them on calls, and sometimes I wonder if, one day, I could leave the control room and go to work as a paramedic. I don't know if I would be any good at it – aside from my disastrous attempt at learning to drive I am very squeamish about broken bones, and I think I might squeal if I saw a leg pointing the wrong way. I'm not very good with vomit either. Every time I smell it I want to add to it. But we shall see! Either way, it's going to be a really exciting day out!

The next morning, I took the new suit I'd bought back to the shop and got my £100 back.

# Hitler Makes an Emergency Call

19 September 2005

Me: AMBULANCE SERVICE, WHAT IS THE ADDRESS OF THE EMERGENCY?

Him: ENGLAND IS RUBBISH. YOU ARE RUBBISH. YOU AND YOUR RUBBISH AMBULANCE SERVICE. I AM HITLER!

Me: ER ... OKAY. DO YOU NEED AN AMBULANCE? IF SO, WHAT IS THE ADDRESS?

Him: I NEEDED AN AMBULANCE, BUT YOU DID NOT SEND ME ONE. HIGH ROAD. NOVEMBER THE SEVENTEENTH. I AM HITLER.

Me: WHAT'S THE FULL ADDRESS?

Him: YOU ARE DAFT! DO YOU SPEAK ENGLISH? DO YOU SPEAK ENGLISH? I AM HITLER. YOU ENGLISH ARE RUBBISH. I TOLD YOU, HIGH ROAD. NOVEMBER SEVENTEEN. I CALLED TWO WEEKS AGO, AND NO ONE SENT ME AN AMBULANCE.

Me: BUT NOVEMBER THE SEVENTEENTH WASN'T TWO WEEKS AGO! IT'S SEPTEMBER – AND IN ANY CASE, I CANNOT ANSWER QUERIES ABOUT AMBULANCES THAT DID NOT COME TWO WEEKS AGO. YOU NEED TO TRY THE COMPLAINTS DEPARTMENT. THEIR NUMBER IS –

Him: YOU ARE RUBBISH! YOUR COMPLAINTS DEPARTMENT ARE RUBBISH! I AM HITLER! ICH HABE EINE BLAUE SIRENE AUF MEINEM KOPF, ABER DAS GRÜNES KREUZ AUF MEINER SEITE IST MIT EINEM SWASTIKA ERSETZT WORDEN! (THIS ISN'T WHAT HE ACTUALLY SAID, I DON'T KNOW WHAT HE SAID BECAUSE I CAN'T SPEAK GERMAN. THE ONLY WORD I UNDERSTOOD WAS 'SWASTIKA' AND APPARENTLY THE GERMAN FOR SWASTIKA ISN'T 'SWASTIKA' BUT 'HAKENKREUZ' SO I SUSPECT HE WAS MAKING IT UP ANYWAY. HE SOUNDED ABOUT AS GERMAN AS THE QUEEN.)

Me: I'M SORRY, SIR, I DON'T SPEAK GERMAN. FRENCH, GREEK OR
    SPANISH, BUT NOT GERMAN. THEY MADE US CHOOSE AT GCSE LEVEL,
    YOU SEE. NOW, IS THERE ANYTHING I CAN DO TO HELP YOU?

Him: KILL THE JEWS! CAN YOU KILL THE JEWS FOR ME?

Me: I'M AFRAID THE MURDER OF JEWS CONTRAVENES LONDON
    AMBULANCE SERVICE POLICY, SIR. PERHAPS YOU WOULD LIKE
    AN AMBULANCE? WE HAVE PLENTY OF THOSE.

Him: YES, I NEED AN AMBULANCE. ONE OF YOUR RUBBISH ENGLISH
    AMBULANCES. ICH BIN DREIZEHN JAHRE ALT UND ICH MAG DIE
    FLÖTE SPIELEN!

Me: WHERE DO YOU WANT THE AMBULANCE TO COME TO?

Him: HIGH ROAD. NOVEMBER SEVENTEEN.

Me: BUT IT'S SEPTEMBER!

Him: NOVEMBER SEVENTEEN! TOTTENHAM! (AT LAST IT DAWNS ON ME
    THAT NOVEMBER SEVENTEEN IS A POSTCODE AND NOT A DATE.)

Me: AND WHY DO YOU NEED AN AMBULANCE?

Him: I HAVE KILLED SOMEONE. HERE. WITH MY BARE HANDS, BECAUSE
    I AM HITLER. ICH MAG GESCHLECHT MIT ZIEGEN HABEN! I KILLED
    THEM HERE, A FEW HOURS AGO.

Me: (ENTERING STANDARD PROTOCOL QUESTIONING IN A DEADPAN KIND
    OF WAY.) ARE YOU WITH THEM NOW? YES? HOW OLD ARE THEY? ARE
    THEY CONSCIOUS? ARE THEY BREATHING?

Him: YOU WANT TO KNOW HOW OLD THEY ARE? WHY? DO YOU FANCY
    THEM? YOU WANT TO DO IT WITH THEM? WELCHE WEISE IST DIE
    STATION, BITTE? YOU'RE A KINKY LITTLE DEVIL, YOU. BUT DAFT. AND
    RUBBISH. THEY'RE A HUNDRED YEARS OLD.

Me: OKAY, AND YOU WANT AN AMBULANCE BECAUSE YOU'VE KILLED
    THIS PERSON. SEVERAL HOURS AGO.

Him: NO, I WANT AN ICE CREAM. WILL YOUR AMBULANCE CREW BRING
    ME AN ICE CREAM?

Me: I'M AFRAID WE DON'T CARRY ICE CREAMS, SIR.

Him: RUBBISH! GEBEN SIE MIR MEIN CORNETTO, KÖSTLICHE EISCREME AUS ITALIEN! LAST TIME THE AMBULANCE CAME, THEY BROUGHT ME ICE CREAM.

Me: I HIGHLY DOUBT THAT, SIR. PERHAPS YOU CONFUSED 'AMBULANCE' AND 'ICE CREAM VAN'. THEY ARE OF SIMILAR SIZE AND SHAPE, BUT ONE HAS A BLUE LIGHT ON TOP WHILE THE OTHER, ER, DOESN'T. IN ANY CASE, YOU APPEAR TO BE WASTING MY TIME. I HAVE YOUR ADDRESS NOW, SO I'M SURE WE'LL BE SENDING YOU SOMEONE. IF YOU WISH TO ENQUIRE ABOUT THE AMBULANCE THAT DIDN'T TURN UP TWO WEEKS AGO, I SUGGEST YOU TRY THE COMPLAINTS DEPARTMENT ON 020 7 –.

Him: RUBBISH. I AM HITLER, AND I SHALL NEVER PHONE YOUR RUBBISH AMBULANCE SERVICE AGAIN.

Me: WE CAN ONLY HOPE, SIR.

# Sally

27 September 2005

I spent twenty minutes on the phone to one of our regular callers tonight. Sally Wiltshire is twenty-four years old and lives above a kebab shop in an insalubrious area of inner London. Just like Brenda her address is tagged on our computer system. The tag reads as follows.

Sally Wiltshire, d.o.b. 20/10/80, alcoholic and psychiatric patient. Has been known to place razor blades in vagina, slashes arms and throat and has previously thrown herself in front of cars. Carries knives. Violent and unpredictable. Send police.

This makes Sally sound like a really unpleasant individual, but believe me, she isn't. I don't know what the ambulance crews would say about her, but to us call takers she is the kindest and most polite individual you could ever come across. She's well spoken and intelligent, and I wonder what could possibly have happened to turn her life into such a mess.

'What's wrong, Sally?' I asked. 'Tell me exactly what's happened ...'

'I've hurt myself ... again ...' sobbed Sally. 'I've cut my arms and my throat and, oh God, I shouldn't have. I'm so stupid! Here I am, wasting your time again. Sorry, sorry, sorry.'

'Don't be sorry,' I told her. 'It's what we're here for.'

I ran through the triage questions, which I'm sure Sally knows by heart. She doesn't flinch when I ask if she's violent or has any weapons. Her answer is always the same – she's only violent to herself, and she has knives and scalpels, but she'd never use them on anyone else. She knows, though, that we won't come to her without the police, and she accepts that. Apparently it's because of 'the incident, that thing that happened when I wasn't in my right mind'. I didn't ask what it was or point out that she's not exactly in her right mind now. I can only assume that she lashed out at a member of the emergency services. I can't believe she'd ever seriously want to hurt someone – she seems sad, not angry.

Believe it or not, Sally is on the road to recovery. Her turning point came with her last suicide attempt, when she deliberately ran out in front of a car on a dual carriageway. She was in intensive care for a month with two broken legs and a crushed pelvis. There was severe internal damage to her liver and spleen and she very nearly died. The doctors told her that her liver was so badly damaged, if she carried on drinking alcohol she would die.

'Have you stopped drinking?' I asked her.

'I can't,' said Sally. 'I've tried. I used to drink two big bottles of vodka every single day, and now I only have one of the little ones.'

'That's good!' I said. 'Well done! You'll soon be off it entirely.'

Sally says nothing. She just cries.

'They said ...' she starts eventually. 'They said that if I carry on drinking, I won't live to see my twenty-fifth birthday. It's a month away, and I haven't stopped. I'm going to die. I don't really want to die. I just want the pain to stop. I just want to stop being so stupid.'

'I don't think you're stupid,' I said. 'And I think that the fact that you've survived all your suicide attempts and not died from drinking when the doctors said you would means something. Maybe you're not supposed to die.'

I heard the doorbell ring in the background.

'Sally? It's PC Duncan here! Open up!'

'Oh hi, Paul!' sniffed Sally, who was obviously familiar with half the local police force. 'Coming! I've got to go now. Thanks for talking.' And she hung up.

I hope Sally gets better. I hope she stops drinking. She sounds such a nice person. She doesn't deserve to die. I don't want to be there when the call comes in to say she's dead.

# One Under

4 October 2005

Two per cent of callers to the London Ambulance Service are hysterical. This figure was drummed into us at Nee Naw Training School. What they didn't tell us was that only about 2 per cent of hysterical callers actually have something worth being hysterical about. When a hysterical caller comes on line (and boy, do they come on line, screaming over the operator's voice as the call is connected and making me jump out of my seat and pull my earpiece away from my ear as I reach for the 'volume down' button) my first thought is, 'Oh, here we go. Cut finger? Toothache? Crying baby?'

This woman actually had something to be hysterical about. She'd been waiting for a train at an open-air tube station on the outskirts of London and, just as the train was pulling into the station, the teenager standing next to her had, for no apparent reason, keeled over and fallen, as if in slow motion, on to the train tracks, right into the path of the oncoming train, and had now disappeared from view. I had to get her to repeat that about seven times, at first all I could hear was 'child under a train, oh my God, oh my God'. It was hard to get a location or anything else out of her – she wasn't entirely listening to me, although not in the usual manner of the Caller That Does Not Want To Listen, more in the manner of someone who is so utterly shell-shocked that the dispatcher's voice just becomes a meaningless squeak in the whirl of horror that is all around them.

Then there was a noise, which could possibly have been the train moving, and the woman said something like, 'I see him!' and then screamed and hung up the phone. I would normally ring back a caller who had hung up, but in this case I saw no point: it was the highest priority of call – HEMS, two ambulances, an FRU and a duty officer were already on the way – and this was one of those cases where the dispatcher is utterly impotent. We can't suggest that people start jumping on the tracks and hauling the patient to safety, after all!

Miraculously, this story has a happy ending. The patient, who turned out to be a teenage girl, had fallen because she had had an ill-timed epileptic fit, but she had somehow managed not to be hit by the train when it went over her. She had injuries to her arms and legs, but was fully conscious and was taken to the nearest hospital by ambulance. I expect she'll be fine.

# Creative First Aid

9 October 2005

Contrary to what you might think, when a caller announces that they are a first-aider, my heart often sinks, the problem being that 'first-aider' can mean anything from 'knows how to put on a plaster' to the members of St John Ambulance and Red Cross who practise first aid all the time, are probably better at it than I am, and could resuscitate a plastic mannequin in their sleep. Since there is no real way of ascertaining the skill level of a first-aider quickly, I tend to act as if they don't know anything and give them all the instructions I would give an untrained person. This is probably very annoying to those first-aiders who don't need to be told – and I apologize if you are one of them – but nonetheless it is better to give instructions that aren't needed than not to give those that are. I hope the following call will serve to illustrate this point.

A group of friends was walking along a canal in Islington and found a man ('probably a junkie!') blue in the face and unconscious on the canal bank. Five of them decided to get on their mobile phones and call ambulances, yelling 'GET HERE QUICK! HE'S DEAD!' (because, obviously, the more calls we get, the bigger emergency it is, and the quicker the ambulance will come) while one of them, who had done a first-aid course when he was sixteen, leapt into action and did resuscitation. After getting the vital details I, the lucky call taker, tried to establish that the self-nominated first-aider was doing everything right – not an easy task when his five friends were all getting worked up.

'Listen here,' said my caller, pompously, 'he's a qualified first-aider, you know. Just leave him to it and send the ambulance!'

I explained patiently (I do a lot of this – 'patiently' gets harder and harder) that the ambulance is already on its way (the Forbidden Phrase!) and my job is to help them look after the patient while they are waiting. After I'd bellowed repeatedly at the caller, asking him to tell me exactly what 'resuscitation' the friend was doing, he lost his temper and shouted, 'He's got him on his side, he's thumping him on the chest and another person is pouring water on his face!'

Not quite what you're supposed to be doing, you see.

I told the caller that that was all wrong, and finally he took some notice of me, took charge of the situation and yelled at his friend, 'OI! YOU'RE DOING IT WRONG! STOP THUMPING HIM!'

Suddenly everyone was the picture of compliance and we got the man on to his back, checked in the mouth, opened the airway and then checked for breathing. Much to everyone's surprise, the man was breathing. Perhaps if they had really known their first aid, they would have checked this small detail before starting their haphazard resus. Still, at least they didn't do proper CPR, because CPR done properly will most likely break the patient's ribs.

I impressed on them that there was to be no more thumping or water over the head until the ambulance arrived and that everyone was just to stand back and let one person keep the patient's airway open and watch his breathing. We had no more trouble until the ambulance arrived, although the caller did start crying into the telephone.

# Brenda Again

15 October 2005

Brenda Kramer was back on the phone today. She was absolutely hysterical.

'Help me, lovey!' she exclaimed. 'The house is on fire! I'm going to die!'

Remembering how I was taken in by her 'stroke' last time, I was somewhat more cynical this time. I noted how there was no commotion or sounds of burning in the background. I noted that none of the other call takers were receiving calls about a fire. I noticed how she'd requested an ambulance, not the fire brigade. None of this made any difference to how I treated the call, though. Never judge the integrity of the caller, we're taught. We called the police and fire brigade, we sent two ambulances and a manager, I stayed on the line and issued platitudes right up until the very second the fire crews turned up, knocked on Brenda's door and were greeted by a distinct lack of burning and the sight of Brenda laughing raucously at her own prank.

I said many things to myself, but none of them were repeatable.

# How to Call an Ambulance

20 October 2005

Easily the best example of this from today's calls would be the elderly wife and 7-year-old granddaughter of a 70-something-year-
old gentleman with multiple lung problems, who unexpectedly
collapsed and stopped breathing at home in front of their very eyes.
The first three minutes after someone stops breathing are critical,
and it's fairly uncommon to get a call within that all-important
window, so when I do, I try to waste no time at all starting CPR.
Unfortunately, neither a disabled seventy-something nor a small
child is great at this (CPR is more strenuous than it looks, and
really hard on the knees!) so I wondered what we were going to do.
I've had healthy twenty-somethings, nurses and care home staff fall
to pieces in the face of the non-breathing casualty and a common
attitude is, 'I might not do it right, so I won't do anything.' This is
terribly frustrating for me, knowing that anything is better than
nothing and that even if the ambulance arrives in half the time the
government says it should, that will probably still be too late.

But this supergran didn't say anything like that. She bounded
over to the other side of the room, with the aid of her magic walking stick, and tried to get her husband flat on his back on the floor,
as per CPR instructions. Meanwhile, the granddaughter picked up
the phone on her gran's instructions, and I heard a faint snivelling.

'Hello,' I said, and asked the child her age. I didn't hold out too
much hope when she said she was seven, but she was the only person there, so I ploughed on. 'I'm an ambulance person and we're
going to help your granddad. There's an ambulance on its way to
you now but we need to help him before it gets there, so I need
you to be really brave for me.'

'Okay,' said a little voice, 'what do I do?' And the snivelling stopped. Just like that. This never happens with adults.

'Tell me what Granny is doing.'

The little girl told me that Granny was trying to get Granddad on to the floor, but not getting very far. She then described that Granddad was on the sofa, so I told her to shout out to Gran –

'Granny!' she said authoritatively. 'Ambulance lady says just get him on his back on the sofa, as flat as you can. No, flatter, Granny!'

Next I got the little girl to tell me every time Granddad took a breath. From this I could determine that his breathing was not totally absent, but following the agonal pattern, which is not really breathing but what happens as someone is dying. It is also easier to reverse than the state of not breathing at all.

I wondered what was going to happen with the next bits of the instructions: they're not designed for seven-year-olds, after all, but the little girl did not seem to care that she had no idea what I was talking about. Granny did the CPR for a good minute or two, without stopping, complaining or asking where the ambulance was. Then I saw on the log that the ambulance was pulling up outside, so I sent her out to meet the crew.

Somewhat voyeuristically, I like to stay on the line for a couple of minutes after the ambulance arrives, if it's quiet enough, and listen to what's going on. In this case I heard the pitter patter of London Ambulance Service steel-toed boots, the rustle of bag and mask, and suddenly our little heroine burst into noisy, childish sobs now that she didn't have to be a brave grown-up any more.

This story has a tentatively happy ending. The man was taken to hospital and was actually breathing at the time. I imagine whatever our wonderful ambulance crew did when they got there got him breathing again, but if it hadn't been for the co-operation and calmness of this unlikely duo, I don't think they would have been able to do anything. Who knows if the man lived another hour, another day, another month or another year? But however long he lived, his wife and granddaughter should feel proud that they overcame their fears and the physical barriers to give him the best chance of survival.

# Team-building Exercise Goes
# Horribly Wrong

28 October 2005

A woman rang from a wine bar in central London to say that another woman had been drinking for about seven hours and had now passed out and soiled herself. This would be bad enough anyway, but it transpired that the defecating lady was the caller's boss. How the boss will ever manage to look her employee in the face again is beyond me.

Time for resignation or relocation, I say.

# Bird Flu

29 October 2005

Me: AMBULANCE SERVICE, WHAT IS THE ADD–
Her: HELLO, I WANT INFORMATION ABOUT BIRD FLU!

Me: PARDON?
Her: BIRD FLU! TELL ME ABOUT BIRD FLU!

Me: I'M SORRY, THIS IS THE AMBULANCE SERVICE. WE DON'T
GIVE OUT INFORMATION ABOUT BIRD FLU, OR ANYTHING ELSE
FOR THAT MATTER.
Her: WELL, CAN I HAVE THE NUMBER FOR BIRD FLU INFORMATION,
THEN?

Me: I'M AFRAID I DON'T HAVE IT.
Her: TSK!
*Click*

# Little Mo

1 November 2005

A young woman rang in floods of tears. I had to get her to repeat what had happened several times.

'My boyfriend [sob] hit [sob ... sob] iron [sob].'

At first I thought she was saying that her boyfriend had hit her with the iron, but after the third repeat I realized that what she was saying was that her boyfriend had been beating her up and that she had grabbed the iron and smashed him over the head with it. It was just like what Little Mo did to Trevor in *EastEnders*. He was now prostrate on the floor, semi-conscious and bleeding, and thankfully – unlike Little Mo – this girl had done the right thing and dialled 999. She was now the model caller, doing everything she could to help her boyfriend, stemming the bleeding with a towel, making sure his airway was clear, lovingly reassuring him that he would be okay and that help was coming. Yet she was the one that had put him there in the first place!

I had mixed emotions. On one hand, it could be seen as self-defence. But hitting someone with an iron to defend yourself, quite frankly, is overkill. A swift kick to the undercarriage can deter a man without endangering his life. This, to me, seemed more like retaliation than self-defence. Some people might think, 'Oh, it serves him right,' but would they say that if a woman punched her male partner and he reacted by nearly killing her?

It's a good job we are supposed to be non-judgemental and not express an opinion. I wouldn't have known which opinion to express.

# Ambulance Games

Night shifts this week. I wish I didn't have to do night shifts. If it wasn't for the fact that a sizeable amount of our pay is unsocial hours allowance, I would drop them entirely. For a start, I'm not very good at staying awake. The call rate really starts to drop around 2 a.m. and you can be waiting fifteen minutes for a call to come in. Staring at a blank, blue screen, my eyes really start to swim. Sometimes I physically can't stay awake. Management have ordered the heating to be turned down late at night, in the hope of the cold keeping us awake, but it doesn't work – it just makes me feel drowsier. Of course, as soon as the beep goes off in my ear to alert me to the fact that a call is coming in, I'm wide awake again. Sometimes I'm halfway through getting the address before I know where I am or what's going on. I never thought when I started this job that I'd be able to take a 999 call on autopilot, but now, after fifteen months, I can.

This week has been especially tough because Management have introduced a new rule – no books or magazines in the control room at any time. Books and magazines were the only things keeping us awake during night shifts, but they are now strictly forbidden as they are distracting and make the place look untidy. All we are allowed to read is work-related material, and – believe me – *Ambulance Today* got a bit dull after my third read of it. EMDs, however, are ingenious creatures, and the following are amongst the games I have seen people playing as an alternative.

- *Ambulance Bingo* – Write nine common ambulance scenarios on a piece of card. For example: 'Old woman fallen out of bed'; 'Caller says, "I don't know, I'm not a doctor!"'; 'Hung up on more than three times in one call'; 'Chest pain'; 'Flu'; 'Embarrassing sexual accident'; 'Caller wants number for Pizza Hut'; 'Caller does not understand English but refuses interpreter'; 'Drunk lying on pavement'. Tick each off as they occur. First person with completed card wins a banana.

- *Guess the Ailment* – Attempt to work out what is wrong with your next caller before they tell you. I am very good at this and can sometimes guess correctly before the caller even speaks. Stomach aches can be identified by a snivelling tone and the caller telling you, 'It's very urgent.' Heart attacks usually begin with the line, 'I don't want to bother you, but ...' If the caller is speaking very fast, it is usually a road traffic accident.

- *Ambulance Call my Bluff* – Steal the medical dictionary from CTA and pick obscure words from it. Make colleagues guess what they mean. Extra fun if you choose rude words.

- *Use the Word* – One call taker picks a word at random, other call takers have to somehow work this into their next 999 call. Words increase in difficulty as the game progresses. Words used last night include headache, cat, blancmange, Newham General, Smirnoff and Lactobacillus casei Shirota. NB: For the sake of retaining one's job, it is best to refrain from playing this game if you are speaking to someone who actually has something seriously wrong with them. Legend has it that one EMD once answered the phone 'Washing Machine Service, what's the address of the emergency?' only to find the call was a cardiac arrest.

# Endurance Record

## 11 November 2005

I have just been on the phone for one hour and fifteen minutes to a crazy young woman who was convinced a half-woman, half-man beast (with no face or legs) and a huge machine of unspecified purpose were waiting outside her door to kill her.

I am sure the dispatch desk deliberately held off sending the ambulance just to spite me.

# Full Moon

12 November 2005

There must be a full moon because all the psychiatric patients have been coming out in force. First of all, Brenda Kramer was on the line complaining of chest pain, cold sweats, difficulty in breathing and pain down her left arm. If I hadn't known better, I would have been convinced she was having a heart attack. I still categorized it as if it were a heart attack, but I am wiser now – I knew she was putting it on. As I suspected, she sent the ambulance crew away after calling them some choice names. Doesn't she have anything better to do than call us?

A few hours later I took a call from Sally Wiltshire. It took a while for me to realize who it was because she was crying and groaning so much that I couldn't understand her. It was only after I'd made her repeat the address five times that I recognized part of it and asked, 'Is that Sally Wiltshire?' Sally seemed really pleased that I knew her name, and stopped crying for long enough to explain what was wrong. She hadn't self-harmed this time – she was in pain from her old injuries sustained at the time she'd been run over. The previous suicide attempt, coupled with the constant alcohol abuse, had ravaged her liver, sending spasms of pain through her body.

'Please stay on the line with me until the police get here,' said Sally. I was happy to do so. Half an hour of Sally is infinitely preferable to the five or six bellyaches and flus I could take in that time.

'You're always so nice to me,' said Sally. 'No one else is nice to me. I bet you wouldn't be nice to me if you saw what I looked like. I'm a hideous monster. I've got scars across my neck and arms from self-harming. My teeth have fallen out from the drink. My skin's a funny colour because my organs are packing up. I'm falling apart. I'm twenty-five years old, but I look and feel eighty-five.'

'Twenty-five!' I interjected. 'You had the birthday the doctors said you wouldn't live to see, then? How's the giving up drinking going?'

'I'm still cutting down,' said Sally. 'I haven't drunk for ... three days now. I spent the money I saved on lottery tickets.'

'And what are you going to buy if you win?' I asked her, thinking she might opt for a house in a nicer area, an exotic holiday, maybe even plastic surgery to hide those scars she hated.

'Nothing,' said Sally. 'There's only one thing I want, and money can't buy that. I want some friends, but no one would ever want to be my friend. I'd give it all to you lot at Ambulance Control, so you wouldn't have to work any more, and you wouldn't have to sit up all night talking to morons like me!'

'That's really kind,' I said. 'But I like my job, and I like talking to people like you. I really hope you find some friends. You deserve them.'

The police came then. I hope Sally will be okay. I wish I could send her some friends as well as an ambulance. But we don't stock friends, just oxygen cylinders and bandages, and I suspect she's seen enough of those.

# Asleep on the Job

13 November 2005

A call taker from A Watch has been suspended for falling asleep on the job! Apparently a call came in and she didn't wake up, and all the caller heard was snoring!

A memo came round from Management today, informing us of their decision to repeal the 'no books or magazines' rule between midnight and 7 a.m. Thank God for that! The rest of the time we are too busy to read anyway, so this is effectively back to square one.

# Death – There, I Said the Word

22 November 2005

Isn't it funny how people are scared to say words connected with death? Here are some examples of what callers have said to me on finding a deceased body.

'I think the worst has happened.'

'He's not conscious ... quite the opposite.'

'He's lying face down on the bed.'

'She's on the floor and isn't moving.'

'He's very cold and blue in the face.'

'She's gone all black and smells bad.'

'He seems to be very seriously injured.'

'He's been very depressed lately ... I think he's cut himself or something.'

The latter case was the biggest understatement I had ever heard. It turned out that the patient had slashed his wrists, taken an overdose and then hanged himself. The ambulance crew reported that the room had blood running down the walls and was like a scene from a horror movie. The 'very seriously injured' man, meanwhile, was found approximately fifty metres from his head after a run-in with a pillar while on his motorcycle.

Despite dealing with death on a daily basis the Ambulance Service are equally reticent about using words such as 'death' and 'dead'. There are actually specific pieces of ambulance jargon to get round ever having to use them. The first of these is the gloriously optimistic 'suspended', which refers to a patient who is unconscious and not breathing but who might return to life. All non-breathing patients are presumed to be in this state until the caller says otherwise, and we call takers waste no time in getting the CPR started, doing everything we can to coax the caller into doing it.

'Purple', on the other hand, refers to a patient who is d-e-a-d. In most circumstances when someone has not been breathing for three minutes, they are beyond resuscitation and thus 'purple' (which, incidentally, is just a randomly chosen code word and not a description of the colour of their face). If a caller thinks the patient has been like that for some time, or if they're cold and stiff, or even starting to decompose (yuck!), then we put 'purple' on the ticket rather than 'suspended' – which lets the crew prepare themselves for comforting bereaved relatives rather than whipping out their bags and masks. In these circumstances we still offer the resuscitation instructions, but it's very much an *offer* and not necessarily one we're hoping the caller will take up. The reason for this is in small part 'just in case' and in large part letting the caller feel they did all they could.

'Purple plus' is what we call a patient who is definitely dead. We usually only make this kind of assertion when the crew have turned up and been greeted with a corpse. I've noticed that other call takers are very jumpy about declaring a patient to be dead, even with such a glorious array of euphemisms to choose from. Even if they dare to write 'purple' or 'suspended', it's usually prefixed with a '?', as if writing that the patient has died on the ticket will increase the likelihood of this being the case. Sometimes, when feeling slightly delirious from lack of sleep, I feel like marking my tickets with 'DEAD' instead of one of these namby-pamby euphemisms, and sending it off like that, in all its unadulterated starkness.

My first 'dead person' call came about a week into my training, at the point when I was taking calls with my trainer listening to me and giving me the odd pointer. It was just after 8 a.m., and the patient's husband had gone to take her a cup of tea and found something was wrong. Very wrong. He'd called us.

'It's my wife,' he explained. 'I think she's had a stroke or something. I can't wake her up and she's a bit blue in the face. She's just come out of hospital after having a heart attack.'

I ploughed through the routine questions. Is she conscious? No. Is she breathing? *No.* It was the first time I'd ever had that answer.

'Okay,' I said, following the instructions on the screen. 'Place her flat on her back on the floor and remove any pillows ... kneel next to her and check in her mouth for any food or vomit. Nothing? Okay, place one hand on her forehead and the other behind her neck and tilt her head back. Can you hear or feel any breathing? No? Right, I'm going to tell you how to do resuscitation ...'.

I think it was only at this point that he realized his wife was in cardiac arrest.

'But she's still warm!' he protested. Of course, that didn't matter. It only meant that she hadn't been dead a long time. All the more reason to press on with resuscitation.

'Right ... okay ... tell me what to do ...' he said, his voice breaking slightly. I gave him the instructions and he pressed on with them valiantly, even though he was elderly himself and it must have been a huge physical effort. I've practised CPR myself on a Resus Annie (a plastic doll with inflatable lungs) and it is surprisingly hard work.

After about five minutes the ambulance arrived and I heard the crew ask the caller, 'When did you last see her?' More than a year into this job, I now know that this is always the first thing the crew ask when it looks like someone has died. They're assessing whether they should start a resuscitation attempt or set about arranging a doctor to certify the death.

Something that I didn't think about before I started this job is the way the number of deaths varies according to the time of year. In the first week of winter, when the temperature drops noticeably and we all get out our hats and scarves, there seems to be a 'death boom'. I always imagined this was down to old people thinking, 'Time to go now! I've had my last summer and can't be bothered to live through another freezing winter – I think I'll just lose the will to live!' But apparently there is a more scientific reason for it – colder weather means the blood clots more, so people are more prone to heart attacks and strokes. Respiratory infections also increase in winter, usually due to people catching colds or flu. People actually dying from exposure to the cold is comparatively rare, although there are some tragic cases of elderly people who have fallen on cold floors and died of hypothermia before they have been discovered.

In summer we are usually busier, but with less serious calls – more people are outdoors, so they're more likely to have accidents, or faint in the sun, or get drunk and pass out. It's getting cold again now, and the deaths are increasing. I'm averaging four per shift.

My record is seven. I think I must have been sitting in the Unlucky Chair that shift.

# Top Ten Most Pointless 999 Calls
# I Have Ever Taken

24 November 2005

I was chatting to one of the CTA paramedics about timewasters today, which got me thinking about the least-deserving calls I have ever taken. Here they are.

1. 'There's a bee in my front room!' (Had it stung anyone? No. Was anyone there allergic to bees? No. It was a straightforward case of Bee In Front Room ...)
2. 'I've stubbed my toe!'
3. 'I had a dream my friend has been shot. I tried to ring him but no one answered. Can you go round and make sure he is okay?' (It was 2 a.m., I'm not surprised no one answered ...)
4. 'My cat has scratched me!'
5. 'I've just got a new SIM card, and I don't know the number. Could you tell me, please?'
6. 'My boyfriend has a boil on his bottom and can't sit down!' (What made this one worse was the fact that the caller kept ringing back every ten minutes, bemoaning the fact that we hadn't sent an ambulance yet.)
7. 'There's a rat in my kitchen!'
8. 'My child has stuck a pea up his nose!'
9. 'I think I'm going to get an abscess in my mouth!' (He hadn't actually got it yet ... I guess he was thinking that prevention was better than cure!)
10. 'I had an accident last week and was taken to hospital by ambulance. I've just been discharged, and there is blood all over the carpet. Could you come round and clean it up?'

That said, these are not the calls that really get my hackles up. When I joined the LAS, I knew that some people make wildly inappropriate 999 calls. They are relatively few and far between, and rarely cause much inconvenience – they are highly unlikely to get an ambulance sent to them, and often provide a source of amusement for an EMD who was about to doze off during the early-morning lull. (It is, of course, less amusing at busy times when there are callers waiting to get through, and I am certainly not recommending that anyone should make this kind of call for our amusement.)

What really gets my goat is the far more common variety of timewaster, who thinks it is appropriate to call an ambulance out for stomach ache, migraine, toothache, flu and other minor ailments that are really the remit of GPs or pharmacists, or maybe can only be cured by retiring to bed, calling in sick and waiting for the problem to go away. I remember clearly as a child being taught to dial 999 and being told it was only for life-and-death emergencies. I wouldn't have dreamed of calling an ambulance for flu or toothache, and I am reliably informed that twenty years ago no one else did either. Yet nowadays 'ambulance' has become synonymous with 'mobile medical treatment unit' or even 'free taxi to the hospital'. These calls aren't rare, and they have a real impact on the time people with more serious ailments have to wait.

Why do the Ambulance Service send out ambulances to these calls? Well, two reasons. The first is that some callers – especially those who do it habitually – know the 'right' answers to the triage questions. They know that if you mention certain symptoms, an ambulance will come blazing on blues and twos, whereas if you tell the truth, you'll get a call back from CTA. The second is that the Ambulance Service are running scared of being sued. While CTA can and do weed out some of the inappropriate calls by pointing out that a GP or a taxi to A&E would be more appropriate, some people insist that they want an ambulance, and we have no option but to send one. You can imagine the newspaper headlines that would result if that 'stomach ache' turned out to be appendicitis and resulted in a burst appendix while the relatives were trying to persuade us to send an ambulance, and you can bet your life that the papers wouldn't point out that the patient refused to consult a GP (who would have authorized an ambulance straight away), or speculate about what would happen if we sent ambulances to every child with stomach ache.

I think things are getting better – ten years ago there was no CTA and no Green Trucks, so these calls would always tie up emergency ambulances. Now the LAS are working on turning the inappropriate calls into appropriate ones by changing the way we respond to them. While, medically, the lower-priority calls are the patients in the least need, sometimes these patients have financial or social needs, and we can help steer them in the right direction. Crews have a procedure for reporting vulnerable adults and children to Social Services so they can get further help.

There's a long way to go, but I hope in the future we'll be able to help people with low-priority symptoms and never have to worry about the impact this has on life-threatening cases.

# Domestic Violence

10 December 2005

One of the things I love about this job is the way it allows you to practise being a total liar and sucking up to people you don't like in order to get things to go your way. A man rings today because his girlfriend has 'a nasty head injury'. One law of emergency medicine is that if someone tells you what is wrong, but not how it happened, nine times out of ten something dodgy has gone on. (On the tenth occasion they just can't explain it in English.) I ask the man how it happened. He pauses, and his girlfriend can be heard whimpering in the background.

'We were having a bit of an argument, and ... um ... well, I sort of pushed her, and she sort of slipped, and hit her head against the ... um ... table and then the ... er ... door.'

The girlfriend in the background starts to cry.

'I see,' I say in a sugary, it-could-happen-to-anyone kind of voice.

'You're not going to have to send the police, are you?' he asks.

I say a lot of things that don't actually answer the question: 'I'm not the police ... it's my job to get your girlfriend's injuries seen to ... the final decision rests with the ambulance crew ... the most important thing is that she gets help.' These are all true, but at the same time I know the dispatch desk will most likely send the call straight down to the police as soon as they see what I've typed on the ticket ('30-year-old female, fell after being pushed by boyfriend, head inj, ? domestic assault'). Putting a '?' before anything is a great get-out clause, because you're not accusing anyone of anything, merely stating it as a possibility.

I carry on speaking reassuringly and calmly to the boyfriend and hope that his girlfriend isn't going to have any more 'accidents' while they wait for the police, I mean, ambulance, and then say goodbye in a way that conveys the message that I have in no way cottoned on to the fact that his girlfriend didn't fall and quite obviously got those injuries when he punched her in the face.

# Call of the Day

15 December 2005

**Caller:** 'I'VE EATEN TOO MUCH, AND NOW I FEEL REALLY SICK. CAN YOU
DIE FROM EATING TOO MUCH? *CAN* YOU DIE FROM EATING TOO MUCH
IN ONE GO? HOW MUCH WOULD YOU HAVE TO EAT?'

# Vicar Stabbed on Parish Round

17 December 2005

'Ambulance Service, what's the problem?'

'The vicar's been stabbed!'

It sounded like a screwed-up episode of *Father Ted*, but I quickly realized it was no joke.

'He just turned up at my door. He's got a huge knife sticking out of his chest ...' continued the poor parishioner, who had probably been in the middle of watching *EastEnders* when this hullabaloo occurred.

'DON'T PULL IT OUT!' I said. I had just been reading a copy of *Chat* magazine where a clumsy DIY'er had narrowly escaped death after inadvertently shooting himself with a nail gun and attempting to remove it with a pair of pliers, and I know from experience that when people see objects stuck in other people, their first reaction is to pull the object out. This usually does more harm than good. For a start, the knife will cut the patient again on the way out – especially if it has a serrated edge – and secondly, keeping the knife in the wound is a way of plugging it and controlling the bleeding.

NB: If you have already removed a knife from someone, do not put it back in again.

From the quick run-through of the questions I could see this was a proper stabbing, just like it is on TV. I take a lot of calls about stabbings – usually in Romford at 2 a.m. on a Friday night – and most of them are just a small flesh wound sustained in a scuffle. Those that are serious tend to be rung in by someone running away as fast as their legs can carry them, or by someone very drunk and abusive, and so the amount of close-range help I am able to give is limited.

This time it was different, though. I have to give a firm pat on the back to the caller. In all the time I have been working here, I have never come across a more co-operative, sensible, quick-thinking caller than him. There were a lot of things to be done before the ambulance arrived, and he must have grown several extra pairs of hands to be able to do them all. He never once complained or thought it was too difficult. He just got on with it. He should be really proud of himself.

First, he did as he was instructed in order to stop the bleeding (taking off his shirt and wrapping it around the wound, avoiding the knife itself), then he got the vicar down on the floor and raised his legs (treating for shock) and followed my instructions to keep the vicar's airway open as he was fast losing consciousness. He shouted outside for help, and some neighbours came in, which meant one could hold the shirt on the wound and another could keep his airway open. I asked about the location of the attacker – the last thing we want is for the ambulance crew to get stabbed on their way to the call – and the caller managed to ascertain that he'd run away. He then had the bright idea of asking the vicar various questions about what the man looked like, which I imagine would have been very useful to the police. Unfortunately, the vicar was in no state to give much information and, three minutes into the call, he started to convulse. This, obviously, is not a good sign and I was relieved to look at the log and see that an FRU, an ambulance, the police and a HEMS car were on their way. The FRU pulled up at the scene a few seconds later and my job was done, so I hung up and felt very proud of a) the Ambulance Service, for getting help there so quickly (four minutes from the start of the call to the arrival of the FRU), b) myself, for not panicking and for remembering to give all the relevant instructions in the right order, and mostly c) the caller, because it doesn't matter what instructions I give or how fast the ambulance gets there, having a caller who has a grip on the situation is the most important factor in those first vital minutes after the incident.

# Christmas Carols

This year I have really drawn the short straw with day shifts today, tomorrow and Christmas Day and a night shift on New Year's Eve. I didn't have to work New Year last year, but I heard it was really busy. Really, really busy.

Alan has got the hump because I won't be able to spend Christmas Day with him or go to his parents' place in Yorkshire. I won't even be able to go and visit my own parents until January for that matter. Offices everywhere are winding down their activities for Christmas but accidents and illnesses have no sense of seasonal timing.

There was an awful 'dead person' call the other day. I get a lot of 'dead person' calls – they're never nice, but they don't usually upset me. This one, however, was really harrowing. The caller had gone to his mother's house and found her 'not moving, I can't wake her up' and I guessed what was coming next. This wasn't an old woman, she was fifty-one. My world-class CPR instructions were duly administered and I could hear clearly what was going on. A child entered the scene and started screaming and screaming. Anyway, it wasn't any of this that I found upsetting but the fact that the son put the phone down near to what must have been a stereo speaker that was blasting out Christmas carols. The whole thing was like some hideous pastiche job. If it had been on the *Casualty* Christmas episode, we would have said it was far too cheesy.

# Nee Naw Christmas

25 December 2005

**Me:** EMERGENCY AMBULANCE, WHAT'S THE PROBLEM?
**Caller:** I'VE JUST PASSED A MAN ON THE ROAD. HE APPEARS TO
HAVE FALLEN OUT OF HIS WHEELCHAIR AND HE'S GOT BLOOD
ALL OVER HIS FACE.

**Me:** ARE YOU WITH THE PATIENT NOW?
**Caller:** NO, I CAN'T STOP – I'M ON MY WAY TO CHURCH AND IT'D
MAKE ME LATE . . .

I started the day in a bad mood. The call from the man on his way to church who couldn't even be bothered to stop and help the disabled man who'd fallen out of his wheelchair rather set the tone as far as callers were concerned. Their attitude was: 'Not only has my inconsiderate relative gone and ruined Christmas by having this fit/diabetic hypo/heart attack, I have to talk to a bloody call taker to get an ambulance! They can't ask me all these questions on CHRISTMAS DAY!' I felt a bit like telling them to bog off and pointing out that we are giving up our Christmases to help people like them, so they could at least be polite. A grand total of two callers wished me a 'Happy Christmas' all day: the nurse from NHS Direct and a homeless man in a call box in Aldgate. The latter saw HEMS fly past on its way to a five-car pile-up on the M4. He thought it was Santa on his sleigh. I didn't have the heart to set him straight.

Much to my disappointment no one had a comical festive accident involving Santa costumes, turkeys or reindeer antlers in unfortunate places. The closest I got was a man who nearly amputated his finger cutting the turkey.

On the plus side, at around 11 a.m., Management came round

with free Sainsbury's mince pies. This raised my spirits sufficiently to allow me to think of rude callers as existing in a parallel universe where it is not Christmas. The genuine callers did take on a new air of poignancy, as if nothing bad was ever supposed to happen at Christmas. I felt myself welling up at the call from a man whose 4-months-pregnant wife appeared to be having a miscarriage and the transfer for a 45-year-old man with terminal cancer to a hospice – probably his last ever journey.

Management did their best to keep spirits high, with the exception of one Scrooge-like individual who was seen doling out Late Reports at 7.10, even though the recipients had valiantly battled their way in despite the lack of public transport and being charged triple fare for taxis, and had still been only ten minutes late. There was a raffle, a Secret Santa (I got a bottle of wine and a hot-water bottle – someone knows me too well!), relaxed breaks and a never-ending supply of food. I filled a plate with turkey sandwiches and sausages on sticks, switched my phone to 'Unavailable' and got stuck in. Unfortunately, I was halfway through my plate when I happened to notice that the call taker sitting next to me was taking a cardiac arrest call – for an elderly man who'd choked on his Christmas dinner. The sounds of the CPR instructions bellowing across the room quite put me off my food.

After lunch Steve the paramedic came up to Ambulance Control with a packet of mince pies for us. He'd had a very uncheerful start to the day as he'd gone to a man who'd dropped dead in the back of a taxi on the way to his grown-up children's house for Christmas lunch! Still, at least paramedics are used to this sort of thing – God knows how the taxi driver felt. And I don't even want to think of the effect it must have had on that poor man's children. Imagine waiting and waiting for your father to turn up, frantically ringing round, wondering where he was and then finally hearing the police at the door ...

Steve and I have arranged a date for my observation shift on his ambulance – it's in two weeks' time. It has taken a while to get it agreed with Management and to find a day that fits in with my rota. I hope we get some interesting calls – but preferably not ones involving broken legs or vomit.

2006

# Nee Naw New Year

1 January 2006

I have never felt quite so morose going to work as I did yesterday. While Christmas at work was actually quite fun, New Year was hell. It was just far too busy for us to be able to have any kind of alternative celebration. Also, while you can always 'make up' for not spending Christmas with your nearest and dearest (by visiting on an alternative day and having a Christmas meal and exchanging presents), you just can't replicate New Year – the point of which for me is to go clubbing or to a big party – on an alternative day. Alan nagged me to pull a sickie and go to a party with him but, much as I wanted to, my conscience wouldn't let me. I knew that this was the busiest day of the year for the Ambulance Service and I'd be letting everyone down if I didn't go in.

I was working at the back-up control room in Bow, which is only open on special days – such as New Year – in order to provide more call-taking positions. I chose to work there because it's closer to my home than the main room, but I soon began to regret the decision. It's a cold, drab place in the middle of an industrial estate with no local distractions and not even a hint of Christmas decorations. Being presented with a cooked breakfast at 11 p.m. was supposed to raise spirits, but did little of the sort. No one really wanted a cooked breakfast, but it was that or nothing.

The night started off more quietly than I had expected. Seemingly, everyone was too busy drinking and partying to call 999. I spent the turn of midnight talking to NHS Direct about a two-year-old who had fallen out of a bunk bed. Someone popped a party popper behind my head, which made me totally lose track of what I was saying. Talk about an inauspicious start to the year! It could have been worse, though – the person sitting next to me was giving CPR instructions at the stroke of twelve.

Suddenly, just after midnight, the call rate took off, and grew and grew and grew. It was as if someone had popped the metaphorical cork of 999 calls. Or maybe once the first person had called for their drunk friend, everyone saw the ambulance tearing through the streets and thought, 'That's a good idea, I'll have one of them.' I took one call after another without a break right up until 7 a.m. when I was finally allowed to go home. I didn't even have time to go out and call Alan to wish him Happy New Year. I won't even bother to tell you about the calls that I took, because quite frankly they were all the same: 'My mate's got drunk and has fallen over'; 'My mate's got drunk and has passed out'; 'My mate's got drunk and someone has punched him'. I don't know what possesses people to call when someone is merely drunk, though. What do they think we are going to do? We can pick them up and put them in the ambulance, but they will still be drunk. We can take them to hospital, but they will still be drunk. And in the morning they will be drunk, in hospital and under those horrible bright lights, with a stonking hangover, and you will still have to pay for a taxi to get them home. Unfortunately, you will not have to pay the cleaning bill for when they vomited in our ambulance – but if you had my way, you would.

# Happy 2006

2 January 2006

Thank God. Christmas is over and finally we are getting back to normal. Annual leave is no longer forbidden and the call rate is manageable once more. Alan has just about forgiven me for neglecting him over the entire festive season.

Let's just hope it doesn't snow.

# Duplicate Calls

After the Christmas rush, this week has been very quiet. Quiet, by the way, is a forbidden word in Ambulance Control, because as soon as someone says it, something kicks off and all hell breaks loose. So there I was, feet on the desk, immersed in a leftover copy of *Chat* magazine, gently snoozing in my reclining chair, and someone must have said that word, because in an instant the screen above our heads went from '10 call takers free, no calls waiting' to 'No call takers free, 21 calls waiting'.

Uh oh. My first thought was: 'BOMB!' Although, remembering 7 July, there was not really much of an increase in call rate at the time the bombs went off. As the calls were answered, every single person had Angel Islington on their screens, and all the callers were reporting different aspects of the same incident.

'A man has been hit by a bus.'

'A bus has hit Sainsbury's!'

'There are two taxis smashed up and pedestrians lying in the road everywhere.'

Piecing the bits together, we worked out what had happened. A bus had gone out of control, ploughing into two taxis, two shops and umpteen pedestrians. People had obviously witnessed only parts of the incident and were just telling us what they could see.

In the next 2 minutes we received 43 calls on the incident, which is the most I have ever seen. There must have been people standing next to each other with their mobile phones out, ringing the Ambulance Service. I know people always say, 'It's better everyone calls than no one calls', and that is true to an extent, but I'd also like to point out the damage that can be done from too many calls.

For a start, they jam the phone lines, meaning that other emergencies don't get through. Secondly, some callers – especially those passing in cars or buses – aren't sure of the exact location or what has happened, meaning we sometimes end up with phantom 'incidents' to which we send an ambulance, only to discover they are actually duplicates of existing calls.

Whenever I tell non-ambulance people this, someone is always sure to mention the case of Kitty Genovese, an American lady who was murdered in 1964, allegedly in full view of thirty-eight witnesses, none of whom called the police. I did a bit of research into this myself, and found that the Genovese case has been widely misreported – apparently there were around ten calls made to the police, but the majority of the callers had not adequately investigated what was going on, therefore not giving the police any reason to attend as a priority, and the rest hung up because 'the police were asking too many questions'. This sounds very, very familiar to me. I'd like to ask anyone who is calling 999 to report something they have witnessed to take a little time to do three things. One, find out exactly what has happened, if you can. Two, find out the exact address of the place where the ambulance is needed. Three, ask other bystanders if they have already called. Doing these things might cause a slight delay in you making your call, but they will save time in the end.

As for the call in Angel Islington, we ended up sending half the fleet down there, so the people of north London had to wait a little longer for an ambulance that night, but at least there were no fatalities. And it woke us all up a bit.

# Private Detective

6 January 2006

A man called to say that his wife had rung him to say she was having an asthma attack, then hung up. He knew that she was at her friend's house, and he knew her friend's number, but he didn't know the address. He rang us, hoping that we'd be able to trace the address from the phone number and give it to him, so he could go round and check on her.

'We can trace the address,' I told him. 'I'm afraid I'm not allowed to give it to you because of confidentiality rules, but we can send an ambulance there.'

The caller wasn't happy with this. He didn't want an ambulance, he wanted to go there himself. I suggested he ask the friend whose house it was, but he told me she wasn't there. It didn't make a lot of sense, but I decided to get on with it and trace the address first and ask questions later.

The BT operator traced the address for me and I told the man that we were sending an ambulance to his wife.

'Okay, okay,' said the man, with an air of defeat. 'Ring me as soon as the crew get there, okay?'

As soon as he'd hung up, I went up to the dispatch desk to tell them something just wasn't right about that call and to be careful what they said to the husband if they needed to ring him back, because he hadn't known the address and had just been far too eager to get it.

When the ambulance crew arrived at the address, there was no answer. Dispatch rang the husband back and told him.

'Are you *sure* she is there?' asked the allocator. 'We're going to have to treat this as a collapse behind locked doors if you are, and that will mean getting the police to break the door down.'

'She's there!' said the man. 'But don't bother the police. Just tell me the address. I'll go there.'

The allocator called the police anyway, and two minutes later we got a message back from them.

**LAS: WE HAVE RECEIVED SEVERAL CALLS FROM THIS GENTLEMAN THIS WEEK. HIS WIFE HAS LEFT HIM FOR A THIRD PARTY AND HE IS TRYING TO LOCATE HER. DO NOT DIVULGE ADDRESS. PLEASE CANCEL ATTENDANCE AT LOCATION. POLICE WILL DEAL. THANKS.**

# Observation Shift I

## 7 January 2006

I got up at 4.30 this morning to get myself to Steve's ambulance station, on the other side of London from where I live, for a 7 a.m. start. As I arrived, Steve and his crewmate Barry were busy kitting out the vehicle. I made a mental note of where the vomit bowls were kept and then joined the other crews in the staff room for a cup of tea. As soon as one paramedic spotted my Emergency Medical Dispatcher epaulettes and deduced that I was from Control, there was carnage. It was like being a mouse in a room full of cats. A million and one questions rained on me about why we send them on late jobs and why flu calls always come down to them as category A. I was glad when it turned 7 a.m. and the phone rang. One of my colleagues informed us that there was a call for every ambulance.

Steve asked me what I'd like to see. A 'working' suspended, perhaps? A BBA? Anaphylactic shock? No, I said, I'd like to see a bit of nasty trauma – but not a broken leg, of course.

I was first in the ambulance and leant over the partition to see what was on the MDT screen. (MDT stands for Mobile Data Terminal. It's a computer screen which shows the crews details of the calls they are attending, messages from Control and satellite navigation. Crews can also press buttons on it to update us in Control when they arrive at a call, take the patient to hospital, etc.)

It was a call to the prison. A prisoner had had his throat slit. This is what happens when I'm not careful what I wish for.

Off we went to the prison, where we were met by a vacant-looking security guard who went through an elaborate ritual of opening and closing gates at a snail's pace before ushering us through and pointing wordlessly in the direction of one of the prison blocks. We were just unloading our equipment from the vehicle when we realized he had disappeared without giving us any indication where he was going. We stood around for a good two minutes, wondering what to do next, before a harrassed nurse came running along and told us we were outside the wrong block. So Steve and I picked up the equipment and ran after the nurse while Barry moved the vehicle. Not a great start.

The prison looked alright from the outside, an unremarkable tall brick building not unlike my primary school. There were gardens and a sports yard, making it significantly more attractive than Ambulance Control. Inside the prison was a different matter. Whoever said prisons were like holiday camps never went to this place. It was as cold inside as it was outside (very). A horrid smell filled the air – a mixture of hospitals and school dinners. The cold white walls were unspeakably bleak. We paced along the balcony – one side was lined with cells and I could hear the prisoners shouting or crying or singing to themselves. Some cells had their slats open, and through the letter-box-sized opening you could see they were the size of a cupboard and just as austere as the outside. On the other side, the balcony looked down to the floor below, where a depressed-looking cook was serving depressed-looking prisoners with slices of pappy white bread and a grey-looking slop. Between our floor and the ground floor was a large safety net, presumably to stop prisoners throwing themselves off in despair.

We reached the medical room.

There was blood *everywhere*. I have never seen so much blood. There were pools of it on the floor, up the wall and even on the ceiling. On the couch sat the patient, wearing what must once have been a white T-shirt and trousers. They were now red. Two nurses were holding a compress to the patient's face. The patient was fully conscious and clutching a cardboard vomit bowl, which was also full of blood.

'Let's have a look . . .' said Steve, and the nurses unwisely pulled the compress away from the patient's face. It was the nastiest wound I have ever seen in my life. Even Steve and Barry looked shocked, and they've seen hundreds of nasty traumatic injuries. The gash started on the lower neck and continued to the lower lip. The cut was full thickness and the skin was gaping, revealing bits of fat and muscle and veins and whatever else one has going on inside one's neck. Blood poured from the wound. Even worse, the cut continued through the patient's top lip, and I could see that it was literally split in two, so when the patient tried to talk the two sections dangled separately. Blood was spurting from this wound in pulses, and I understood this meant an arterial bleed. His mouth was filling up with blood and clots, which he kept spitting into a bowl. The thing that struck me about the prisoner was that he just looked like an ordinary lad – I guess I'd been expecting some kind of psycho murderer type with big scary eyes and a cold face, but this was just an ordinary guy like Alan. It wasn't a high-security prison, maybe he was just in there for shoplifting or drink driving. He looked terrified and very, very young. The nurse explained that he'd argued with one of the other prisoners, who'd gone away and fashioned a weapon out of an ordinary razor by removing the plastic, then gone back to our patient and, without warning, slashed him across the face with it.

Steve opened his bag of dressings and bandages and stood looking at it, scratching his head and wondering what on earth to use, before settling on some Steri-Strips and some gauze to hold against the wound. A member of the prison staff came in and told us HEMS was circling overhead – he obviously expected us to know all about it when in fact we did not even know HEMS had been requested. (Usually HEMS is either requested by the crew or automatically sent as soon as the nature of the call is known, but in this case they'd decided to activate it just after we'd left the vehicle.) I came in useful at this point because Steve wasn't allowed to use his mobile to call Control inside the prison and I was the only person who knew the control room's phone number. So I rang the HEMS desk, gave them the medical report and made sure they were able to land (and were met by someone more competent than the guy who'd met us!).

Minutes later two doctors and a paramedic, all wearing bright orange suits, barged in.

'Hello, HEMS!' I said nervously, pointing to my dispatcher epaulettes. 'Control staff! Observing! Don't ask me to do anything! Talk to him!'

'Am I goin' in an 'elicopter?' said the patient, his eyes suddenly lighting up, before his mouth refilled with blood and he went back to spitting in his bowl. He sounded about ten.

And then I stood well back as HEMS, Steve and Barry all did their best to get the bleeding under control with adrenaline-soaked gauze, Steri-Strips, and good old-fashioned Firm Steady Pressure. This didn't stop the bleeding completely, but it definitely slowed down to the point where we could think about transferring the patient to hospital. HEMS decided against taking him in the helicopter to the Royal London. There was a local hospital that specialized in trauma and it would be easier to take him there in the ambulance with HEMS on board. I can tell you, it was a bit of a squash in that ambulance: one patient, one prison guard, two doctors, one HEMS paramedic, Barry driving and me in the front. We took the patient in on blue lights but Barry had to be very careful going over the speed bumps to avoid knocking everyone over in the back!

'Suzi!' hissed Steve, as we disposed of our patient in A&E. 'That's it. I'm not asking you what you want for your next call, and if you do wish for anything, make it a nice little old lady who has fallen over.'

'But I want to see a suspended!' I wailed.

Steve just shot me a filthy look.

'Did you hear why the other prisoner did that to him?' said Barry.

'No,' I said, thinking it must have been something really nasty. It's tough in prison. Drugs, gangs, guns.

'Bread!' said Barry. 'Apparently they had an argument over the last slice of bread. Other guy goes back to his cell, comes out with the razor, and does that. All over a slice of bread.'

I thought back to the piles of pappy bread on the way in, the revolting smell, the sight of the prisoner's lip flapping and the exposed flesh in his neck, and all I could do was shake my head.

\*

Back in the ambulance, as soon as we'd cleared up the blood and finished the paperwork, the MDT rang again. Steve peered over to see what we had this time.

'You know you wanted to see a suspended? Well, we've got you one.'

'Hahaha,' I said, not believing him. 'What is it really?'

'It's a suspended!' said Steve, igniting the blue lights and nee naw sirens and launching the ambulance on to the wrong side of the road.

I looked at the screen and saw he wasn't joking. Then I panicked. Then I said some bad words. Then I turned a bit green.

The call, which was to an '85-year-old male, ? suspended, ? purple, been ill with [this, that and the other]' was about ten metres from an ambulance station, so despite getting there in four minutes, we were the third vehicle on the scene, along with an FRU and another ambulance. It is usual practice to send at least two crews to 'working' suspendeds, because there are various things that need doing, for example, CPR, cannulating, intubating, defibrillating, getting equipment ready and herding upset relatives to a safe distance.

Steve cattle-prodded me into the room, where all six of us proceeded to stand in a line and look at the scene in front of us. The other crews had already established that this was not going to be a working job: the patient was, in ambulance-speak, purple plus. In other words, very obviously dead. I had always imagined that dead bodies would be found lying flat on their backs with their eyes wide open, blank and staring, but this gentleman had instead got himself into a most odd position. It appeared as though he had realized something was wrong in the night and had got up from his bed, then thought better of it and sat down and curled up in a ball where he was, his head resting on the bedside cabinet, his face turned away so you could only imagine his expression. I was grateful for this – I imagined it to be peaceful, as in sleep, but for all I know it could have been grossly contorted, frozen as he cried out in pain. Maybe that's why he didn't want anyone to see it. His skin was waxy and almost white. The FRU woman told us that he'd probably been dead for hours. He'd last been seen at bedtime the previous night and by now rigor mortis had completely 'set in – he couldn't be moved at all. My only experience of death before today had involved various small rodent pets, who generally crawl away and hide somewhere to die, and this gentleman's position struck me as similar. Barry told me it was actually very common to find dead people in that kind of position.

From a call-taking perspective handling suspendeds is very different because, as a call taker, you never give up hope and always act as if something can be done. In no circumstances do you acknowledge that the patient is dead. Even if the caller does not perform CPR, you still have the fact that you are sending an ambulance to fall back on, as if the appearance of the ambulance will somehow make everything alright. Today I had no magic ambulance to absolve me; I was part of that ambulance. As all six of us stood there, doing nothing, a somewhat eerie feeling of ineffectiveness crept over me. As the last crew in we were surplus to requirements and shuffled out to leave the others to deal with the formalities (mainly arranging a GP to certify death) and give the relatives space to grieve. As we left, we encountered the patient's daughter, who was walking aimlessly up and down the corridor clutching a mobile phone and keys. The other crew had already told her that her father was dead. As she saw us leaving – testament to the fact that there was nothing we could do for him – she broke into tears. I didn't know what to say to her, so I told her that I was sorry, feeling that this was an incredibly inane thing to say but still better than saying nothing at all.

Back in the ambulance Steve selected 'Deceased, not removed' as the outcome, then checked to see if I was traumatized or anything by my first encounter with a dead body. I was relieved to find I wasn't traumatized, just that it had been somehow different from what I had expected – the position of the body, the way that he was so obviously dead and that no examination was needed, the feeling of 'what now?' once the certainty of the death was established.

'That's about as good as they get,' remarked Barry. 'Sometimes you find them in pools of vomit, pools of blood or pools of faeces.

Sometimes you find them in pools of all three. Sometimes you find them a week later when their face is moulded into the bedside table. Sometimes you find them when the flies have moved in and the smell won't get out of your hair for a week.'

'Next time,' said Steve, 'we'll find you a working job. Pumping the chest, shocking the heart ...'

'Noooo!' I said. 'Can we please just have nice little old ladies who have fallen over from now on?'

Then it was back into Green Mobile, ready and available for the next call.

# Back to Work

## 8 January 2006

After the excitement of the observation shift it was a bit of a drag going back to work. The dingy, cold control room seemed so oppressive compared with the excitement of blazing along at 60 mph on the wrong side of the road with lights blazing and sirens blaring. The remainder of the day's calls had been less exciting – a baby with flu, a minor RTA, a couple of diabetics and a suspected heart attack that turned out not to be – but the first two calls had been enough for me! I've been thinking ever since about whether I would like to be a paramedic like Steve, and I'm still not sure. Weirdly it's not the danger or the responsibility that worry me, or even the potential for vomit and broken legs. It's the thought of the blue-light driving. Those driving lessons I had back when I was working at the hospital were a disaster. Then again, much to my driving instructor's horror, I frequently broke the speed limit and attempted to drive through red lights or in the wrong lane, all of which are requisites of blue-light driving, so maybe I wouldn't be that bad after all. I don't know.

I think I'll arrange another course of lessons and see how it goes – and badger Steve and Barry to take me out again!

# Maternataxi

15 January 2006

Ambulance crews really hate getting called out to women in labour. Giving birth – unless it happens really quickly, something goes wrong, or there is a specific problem which has caused a medical professional to tell the mother to ring 999 when labour starts – is not a medical emergency. It is a perfectly natural thing that happens to thousands of new mothers every year, and most of these manage to plan some way of getting to hospital. After all, they've got nine months! It really worries me when a mother-to-be tells us that she can't take a taxi because she can't afford one. How on earth is she going to afford a baby? The other excuse that makes my blood boil is, 'I just want to be in the ambulance in case something happens.' Should we park an ambulance outside your house too, just in case your baby happens to get ill? While we give these women their taxi ride to hospital 'just in case' there are people waiting out there who have already broken their leg or had a stroke, and we can't help them.

I appreciate that occasionally the best-laid plans go awry and a woman in normal labour might feel it her only option to call an ambulance – maybe there are no taxis available for two hours, her partner has been called away on emergency business and her friends are all at work, an hour away – but maternataxi calls aren't occasional, and there is never any kind of explanation as to why they can't get there themselves, they simply feel they are entitled to an ambulance. We get a ridiculous number of inappropriate calls for women in labour. Sometimes I even hear a relative on the scene saying they won't go in the ambulance, but they'll follow in the car. So why don't they just drive the patient to the hospital? Who knows? A sense of entitlement or misinformation? Whatever the reason, I wish we could stop it. Apparently there are other ambulance services in the UK who can refuse point blank to send a vehicle to a woman in labour unless there is a genuine emergency.

Unless the woman is having problems or is about to give birth on the spot, most maternataxi calls turn out as green, the lowest priority. This means that a lot of women in labour have a long wait, during which some of them wise up and get in a car. Others ring back every five minutes, shouting at me and saying things such as, 'Do you want me to have my baby right here?' to which it is very difficult not to reply, 'Well, yes – at least then it would be a proper emergency!'

The other day, however, there was a call from a woman who used a special technique to get an ambulance to ferry her to hospital in the early stages of labour. This technique is known as Telling Porkie Pies. As I explained earlier, we have to ask a series of questions (to which we have already guessed the answer) to ensure that we haven't missed anything. In the case of a maternity one of the questions is, 'Can you see, feel, or touch any part of the baby yet?'

'Yes,' replied the woman – the woman in labour, who was talking calmly with no sign of pain or panic in her voice – 'I can feel the head.'

Thinking that she had probably misunderstood the question, I rephrased it, using the word 'vagina' and everything.

'I told you – the head is out!' said the woman.

This put me in a difficult position, because from my (admittedly limited) experience of women giving birth I can tell you that they generally do not talk calmly on the phone while the head is emerging from their vagina. On the other hand – never disbelieve a caller! Expect the unexpected! So I got the caller to summon her sister from the next room, and got the sister to check the vagina, hoping that she would tell me that there was definitely no sign of the head, but instead she told me the same thing: 'Yes, I can see the head.'

There was nothing much I could do except take their word for it and press on with the birthing instructions. I sent the sister off to fetch towels, and she returned to the phone after a suspiciously short length of time. I told her to get the pregnant lady on to the bed in the correct position and stripped off, and she told me that she was already in that position. I then told her to place her palm against her sister's vagina as the baby delivered, and she told me she was doing it. I knew she wasn't. Don't ask me how – we don't have video phones, after all – but I can tell if instructions are actually being followed or if the caller is pretending, every single time. Then I waited. And waited. Of course, the head didn't get any further and during the whole time the mother-to-be made neither a grunt nor a moan. I could hear no evidence of her having contractions, let alone giving birth.

Then there was a buzz at the door and the FRU paramedic burst in, no doubt expecting to see the baby taking his or her first breath, and instead was greeted by a heavily pregnant woman sitting fully clothed on the sofa.

'I thought you said the head was out!' he said incredulously.

'Oh no!' said both women in unison. 'We said that the labour had just started!'

At this point I felt a bit like banging my head on the desk.

# Vicar on TV!

16 January 2006

I was sitting in the mess room watching *London Tonight* when what should come on but an article about the Vicar Stabbing Incident! There it all was in technicolour, stills of the street where it happened, photos of the vicar himself and – best of all – an interview with my caller! I have never been able to put a face to any of my patients before – except the baby from the Leek and Winkle toilets, and all babies look the same to me – so this was just great.

Apparently the vicar is in a 'serious but stable' condition in the local hospital and the assailant has been caught and detained under the Mental Health Act. The caller even referred in his interview to how the Ambulance Service gave him instructions over the phone, and as a concession to his bravery I'm prepared to overlook the fact that he called me 'the operator'.

# One False Step

Elderly people are always falling – out of bed, off the commode, out of their wheelchairs, in the street, on the floor – and their equally elderly partners are always getting in a flap about it, so when an elderly lady's panicked voice came down the line telling me her husband had fallen on the stairs, the 'serious call' sensor in my head failed to be activated. Mental alarm bells only started to ring when she reported that her husband was not responding to her at all. By the time she reported that her husband had started 'snoring', the metaphorical sound was deafening. Within seconds my perception of the call had gone from run of the mill to a highly unusual suspended trauma call. I guessed that, as it is unusual for someone to curl up for a doze after taking a six-foot tumble, the 'snoring' was actually agonal breathing.

When I first started this job, the prospect of identifying a patient as having agonal breathing, and subsequently starting resuscitation on them, really worried me. What if I got it wrong and ended up breaking someone's ribs when they were breathing all along? Luckily a new version of the AMPDS software – what we use to tell us which questions to ask and which instructions to give – includes a 'breath timer'. You get the caller to tell you every time the patient takes a breath, click the mouse when they do, and after five breaths it will tell you if it is agonal breathing or proper breathing. It is a great gadget when it works, but the main impediment is getting your caller to concentrate on telling you when the patient breathes, and nothing else. They tend to deviate and tell you some useless piece of information, missing a breath, meaning you have to start all over again ...

After my third go using this gadget I determined that the breathing pattern was indeed most likely agonal (and I'd ascertained that the patient had broken his hip last year and suffered from angina), so I gave CPR instructions to the old lady. This wasn't easy – she was, understandably, panicking and, as with many elderly callers, she didn't understand that the ambulances are sent out by computer. She kept repeating two of my least favourite phrases: 'Hurry up!' and 'Just send the ambulance!' I felt a bit like retorting, 'I am giving instructions which could save your husband's life, this is not something that should be *hurried* through,' and, 'If I *just* send an ambulance and do nothing else, your husband will undoubtedly be dead by the time it arrives.' But this would have been rude and achieved nothing, so I deliberately paused to check the location of the ambulance on the log and told the old lady what I was doing – an action that served no purpose other than to illustrate the fact that an ambulance was actually coming. I emphasized my point with the Forbidden Phrase, hoping no one would pick up on it. It still didn't work. The next thing out of the old lady's mouth was, 'Tell them to drive faster!' I wanted to say, 'The ambulance crew are driving on blue lights and sirens! They're belting down the wrong side of the road at forty miles an hour! Do you want them to drive even faster and risk crashing and not getting there at all?' I didn't say that either, of course. I took a risk and named the road that the ambulance was coming down – a particular main road a mile or two from her house, something concrete that she couldn't argue with.

Bingo. Finally she believed the ambulance was coming and that I wasn't just fobbing her off. Once she started the CPR, she didn't mention the ambulance again and followed my instructions perfectly for the four minutes or so until the ambulance arrived. I was very careful not to imply that he was dying or 'not breathing' as that would have freaked her out more, but instead told her he wasn't breathing as often as he should, so she would have to give him some extra breaths. She did everything brilliantly and I was very impressed – a lot of elderly people refuse to give CPR because they can't physically do it, not to mention being scared. Fortunately, she didn't have to wait long before the crew burst in like the heroes they are.

Unfortunately, the outlook was not good – the patient was still not breathing when he was rushed into hospital, although I suppose the fact they took him in must have meant they thought he had some sort of chance. In general, though, once someone has stopped breathing from trauma their chances are not good anyway, and his age and the fact that he had stopped breathing within a minute of the accident, indicating a very serious injury – maybe a broken neck? – all counted against him.

This call made me think about how strange and fragile life is – this man was in his seventies, and that morning, as far as I know, he'd been relatively healthy, despite facing all the diseases and dangers the average person would come across in seventy-five years, and was probably expecting to enjoy many years of retirement with his wife before fading out gradually from some kind of age-related illness. And yet, one false step, one piece of loose carpet, one instant not looking at his feet, and his life was over, just like that, in the space of ten minutes.

# Crying Baby

23 January 2006

**Me:** AMBULANCE SERVICE, WHAT'S THE PROBLEM?

**Girl:** MY BABY WON'T STOP CRYING! SHE IS TEETHING!

**Me:** ER, IS THERE ANYTHING *WRONG* WITH YOUR BABY? DO YOU THINK SHE MIGHT BE ILL?

**Girl:** NO, SHE AIN'T ILL! SHE'S TEETHING!

**Me:** SO, LET ME GET THIS STRAIGHT – YOU WANT AN AMBULANCE BECAUSE YOUR BABY IS TEETHING, AND YOU'RE SURE THERE'S NOTHING ELSE WRONG?

**Girl:** I NEED SOME 'ELP 'ERE! SHE WON'T STOP CRYING!

**Me:** OKAY, THEN. (AND I LAUNCH INTO OUR 'CATCH-ALL' SICK PERSON PROTOCOL, WHICH ATTEMPTS TO IDENTIFY IF THE PATIENT HAS ANY OF THE 'PRIORITY SYMPTOMS' WE LOOK FOR, AND CAN SOUND QUITE OBLIQUE AND NONSENSICAL IF THEY DON'T.) IS SHE CONSCIOUS? IS SHE BREATHING? IS SHE BREATHING NORMALLY ...?

**Girl:** WELL, OF COURSE SHE IS! THERE AIN'T NO NEED TO ASK SARKY QUESTIONS!

# Comeuppance for Brenda?

1 February 2006

I took a call from Brenda's house today.

'Help!' said a high-pitched voice. 'It's Miss Kramer ... I think she's been stabbed! There's blood everywhere! I think she's DEAD!'

I sat up in shock. Oh my God, after all those prank calls something really had happened to Brenda. She'd annoyed the hell out of me, but who would want to kill her? She was an institution and, if she really was dead, I was going to miss her ...

'Help is being arranged for you while we're speaking,' I told the neighbour. 'I'm going to ask a few questions and then I'm going to tell you what to do to help her.'

'Thank you so much, lovey!' said the neighbour, her voice dropping an octave.

'Wait a minute!' I said. 'Lovey' is an endearment Brenda often uses. 'Brenda, is that you?'

There was a sharp intake of breath, and the line dropped. Yes, Brenda was impersonating her neighbour and, sure enough, the ambulance crew found her alive and well.

Once again, I'd been taken in. I had to take my hat off to Brenda. She's got hoaxing down to a fine art.

# Child on the Line

Whenever a child dials 999, the operator comes on the line as the call is put through, telling us that they're connecting a call from a child. This is because about 90 per cent of calls from children are the little devils playing with mobile phones. Mums and dads, please keep mobiles out of reach of little hands! On Christmas Day it seemed we spent half the day ringing back mobiles and trying to trace their owners, only to find some small person had got carried away with their new 'toy'.

Anyway, yesterday the operator came on the line telling me there was a call from a child, and then there was silence. I was fully expecting this to be the usual child playing scenario – when children do make genuine calls, they are actually a lot better at it and are calmer than adult callers.

'What's the problem? What's happened?' I said, for the third time, and finally a little voice started to speak.

'Can you come? Mummy's cut her wrists and there is blood everywhere!'

'Oh hell,' I thought, 'not a child playing after all.' (Unless it's one with a really sick sense of humour.)

'Yes, we can come,' I said. 'What's your address?'

'Don't know!' said the child. 'I rang my uncle and he told me not to call you and that if I did I would get in trouble!'

This was just getting worse and worse. I sensed the child was scared to give me her address because of what her uncle had said but, after a bit of coaxing, she provided the name of a hotel, the fact that it was in London and a room number. Unfortunately, she had a bit of a lisp, so when she said 'four thirteen' I thought she said 'floor thirteen' and I asked her for the room number again.

'I already told you, four thirteen! Aren't you listening?' she said indignantly, which would have made me laugh if it hadn't been such a dire situation. Children sound really amusing when they are trying to be authoritative.

'Okay, you're doing really well,' I said. 'Now I just need to know the street name and which part of London it's in – do you know that?'

'No!' wailed the child, breaking into noisy sobs. 'My uncle said you wouldn't come! You're not coming, are you?'

'Yes!' I said, trying not to panic – the sound of a small child in such obvious distress not helping much. 'Of course we'll find you, we'll look everywhere until we do, but if we knew a bit more of the address we'd find you faster.'

'MUUM-MEEEEE!' screeched the child. 'MUUUUUM-MEEEEEEEEEEE! Come here, Mummy! Come here, Mummy!'

Eventually a woman came to the phone and I asked her for the address.

''Salright,' she said in a slurred voice, 'm'okay, jusssht fine. Don' send the umblunce, mmfine.'

'Just let us send someone round to see if you're okay?' I asked, but the phone went down.

Theoretically we are not supposed to send a vehicle to someone who says they do not want an ambulance, because everyone has the right to refuse medical aid, but I decided in this case the child was a 'patient' too, and in just as great need as her mother. I rang the mobile phone company, who found the phone's approximate location from the signal, and also Directory Enquiries. I found the address of the hotel and off went the ambulance and the police.

The ambulance crew got there first and someone, probably the child, let them in. They reported back to us that the patient had been self-harming and was very drunk, and the child was only five years old. This shocked me – I had assumed she was older. I'm useless at telling kids' ages from their voices, and even if they are standing in front of me I am not much better, but from the maturity displayed in her language and the way she took charge of the situation I would have put her at about ten. The patient was refusing to go to hospital, but after the police arrived everything went quiet for a while and then the ambulance set off for the hospital, so she must have changed her mind.

I hope they both got the help that they needed.

I've been thinking about this poor little girl a lot. When I was five, life was all My Little Pony, Care Bears and Morten Harket – and I don't think I knew that self-harming even existed.

# Phantom Appendix

Me:  WHAT'S THE PROBLEM?
Him:  I'VE GOT APPENDICITIS!

Me:  HOW DO YOU KNOW IT'S APPENDICITIS?
Him:  BECAUSE I HAD IT BEFORE! AND I HAD TO GO TO HOSPITAL!
   AND HAVE MY APPENDIX OUT!

Me:  YOU HAD YOUR APPENDIX OUT?
Him:  YES.

Me:  AND YOU THINK YOU HAVE APPENDICITIS?
Him:  YES!

Me:  IN YOUR APPENDIX?
Him:  YES!

Me:  WHICH YOU HAD TAKEN OUT?
Him:  OH ...

# My Baby's Not Breathing

10 February 2006

'My baby's not breathing' is probably number one on the list of 'things call takers don't want to hear'. Unfortunately, it was exactly how the call began.

'Help! My baby's not breathing,' said the panicked mother. 'He's blue and his face is covered in vomit . . . I think he's choked on it!'

I asked for the address immediately. I wouldn't have understood what she said but fortunately she was calling from a landline, so I could see her address. She lived on a dual carriageway. When you get a call to a dual carriageway, it's important to find which carriageway the address is on, otherwise the ambulance may be sent from the wrong direction, meaning it has to go all the way up to the next junction, go round a roundabout and come back. Not a delay you want when you have a non-breathing baby.

The caller lost it. She couldn't remember whether it was east-bound or westbound and quite frankly she didn't care! 'Just send the ambulance! Hurry up! My baby's not breathing. It's an emergency!' I could see it from her point of view – her baby wasn't breathing, and there I was asking stupid questions such as 'What side of the road do you live on?' Of course, from my point of view, the question was vitally important . . . but there was no time to explain why. I got the baby's age – one and a bit – then asked her what had happened. She'd heard a strange noise on the monitor and come in and found the baby like this. Straight on to the CPR instructions. Clean the vomit out of baby's mouth – there was plenty, so it took a while – then tilt the baby's head back and listen for breathing.

I already had the 'Start Compressions' card fired up when the mother told me that actually, yes, the baby was taking shallow breaths.

He was twitching a little bit too, she noticed, but otherwise unresponsive. I let out an audible sigh of relief and gave the mother the instructions for maintaining the airway, while using the 'breath timer' gadget to make sure the baby was breathing regularly. He was. Now there was nothing to do but wait for the ambulance. I decided to ask the mother a few more questions about what had happened (the purpose of these is usually more to distract the caller and make her feel she is doing something than to find out anything important). The baby had been ill with a cold, but didn't have a temperature. She'd heard choking noises on the baby monitor, which is why she'd assumed he'd choked on vomit. When she cleared the vomit from the baby's mouth, his teeth had been clenched and he nipped her finger. It was sounding more and more as if he'd had a fit, so I marked the ticket '? fitting' to make sure a paramedic crew was dispatched.

Just before the first ambulance crew arrived (two had been sent, as is protocol with any 'working' cardiac arrest — although I had confirmed the baby was breathing, no one wanted to take any chances!), I heard a very welcome sound. The baby started to cry! Emergency Medical Dispatchers are the only people in the whole world who like the sound of a crying baby! (I only wish this were still true whenever one sits next to me on the bus.) I bet the crew were relieved to find the baby was alive too. I listened in for a couple of minutes, and what I heard the crew saying confirmed that they also thought the baby had just had a fit. Fits are quite common in babies, and not usually life-threatening, though it is always recommended that you call an ambulance if your baby is fitting. The mother was asked which of the two nearby hospitals she'd prefer to go to, and at this point I'd heard enough and hung up, relieved. They wouldn't be letting her pick and choose hospitals if the baby was in a life-threatening condition. I think he was probably breathing all along and the mother mistook the tail end of a fit for a cardiac arrest. It's also possible that the vomit was blocking his airway, and clearing the airway saved his life — in which case the mother must be thinking that baby monitor was the best investment she ever made! Whatever the case, it definitely felt to me that the baby had come back from the dead.

# 999 Idiot of the Week

17 February 2006

As the phone pinged in my ear to let me know a call was coming in, the mapping screen centred in on the source of the call. The caller was inside a house, approximately one hundred metres from a well-known A&E department in north London.

'This had better be good,' I thought to myself.

It wasn't.

'I've 'urt me arm, riiight!' squawked the caller. 'I wanna get it seen ta!'

'Er, okay,' I said. 'What exactly happened?'

'Well,' explained the caller, 'I stole dis car on Tuesday, riiight, and I was drivin' it orf, and then I saw duh pigs, riiight, and I fort, f*** it, and I got out duh car, but I fell, riiight, an' I landed on me arm, right …'

'Um,' I said. 'I, er, see. So, let me get this straight: you want an ambulance to take you to the hospital, which you live two minutes' walk away from, for an arm injury you sustained three days ago while trying to avoid being arrested by the police?'

'Yeah!!' said the caller. 'Thaz right! So send me a f***ing ambulance, riiight!' And the line went dead.

Put it this way, an emergency vehicle with blue flashing lights was soon on its way to the address, but it wasn't an ambulance …

# It's Not my Job

22 February 2006

The following call was received from a pharmacy on one of the busiest streets in central London.

'Someone just shouted "call an ambulance",' explained the woman. 'There's ... someone bleeding in the road, or something.'

'What's the address?' I ask.

The woman told me that it was outside the address she was ringing from. Checking my 'possible duplicates' screen, I saw that there'd been a motorcycle accident about fifty metres away. I explained this to her, and asked her to go outside and check the location of the patient and find out what had happened.

'Oh no!' said the woman. 'I can't do that, I can't leave my shop. I have customers to serve!'

Nice to see where her priorities lay.

'Okay, can you send someone else?'

'No, there is no one else here!' she said.

'What about the customers you just mentioned?'

The woman muttered something I couldn't hear, and then a young man came to the phone. I tried to ask him to go out and check what was going on, but I didn't get far before he started shouting and swearing at me.

'Look, you bloody timewaster! Stop f***ing asking me to go outside! She's dead, okay! Someone is dead! Send the f***ing ambulance and stop asking stupid questions!'

And then the line went dead.

Now, I've had the 'stupid questions' accusation quite a few times before, and I can understand people getting annoyed with some of the AMPDS triage questions, but I can't believe that someone thinks that knowing the location and condition of the patient is an irrelevancy. Had he stayed on the line, I would have had another 'stupid question' to ask, which would have been, 'How do you know she is dead if you haven't even seen her?'

As much as I'd have liked not to, I had to ring the pharmacy back. This time I got a third person, an older man. I explained to him that someone had rather abusively told me that someone was dead, and that two people had refused to go out and investigate. I explained that at the moment we had two ambulances on their way (one to the accident round the corner, and one to the pharmacy) and that I needed to know if it was the same patient, so that we didn't waste an ambulance. I explained that if she was 'dead', we needed to start CPR, which I could instruct him on, or else she would definitely die. Do you think I had more luck with this man? No, of course I didn't.

'I am not going out!' he huffed. 'I am working!'

'Send someone else, then!' I implored.

'There is no one else!'

'I have spoken to three different people in your shop,' I pointed out. 'Surely one of them can be bothered to step outside the shop in order to help this poor lady who might not be breathing!'

'No!' said the man. 'That is your job!'

'My job is to instruct you as to how to help her. And you,' I said, 'are stopping me from doing my job.'

'I am not a doctor!' said the man irrelevantly. 'I cannot do anything. Goodbye!'

Now, I don't know about you, but I think that helping your fellow human beings is everyone's job, not just the responsibility of those who are paid to do it. Have these people never been in need of help? How would they feel if they were injured and everyone walked past, saying 'It's not *my* job'?

# It's a ... Baby!

## 25 February 2006

Today, I delivered my fourth baby! My first, the one in the pub toilet, was quite dramatic but the other two were fairly anticlimactic and just consisted of someone shouting 'Ambulance, quick! The baby is coming NOW!' and then me shouting instructions into an abyss of people panicking and not listening while the baby delivered itself the way nature intended. This time, however, I really felt like I was helping and playing an active part in the baby's birth.

The call came in around 10 a.m. and was made by the baby's father. The mother was nineteen and it was her first baby, and I guess she thought labour was going to take a lot longer than it did. This makes a change – a lot of first-time mothers dial for a maternataxi as soon as they miss a period. Still, there was no time to discuss why they weren't at the hospital yet, as the baby was well on its way. The father-to-be reported that there was 'some kind of THING!' appearing 'down below' and howled that he needed an ambulance really quickly.

'Sorry, mate,' I said, 'but it looks as if we're going to have to deliver this baby now. The ambulance is coming, but I doubt it'll make it in time.'

'But I don't know what I'm doing! I'll have to cut the cord and stuff and I don't know how!' wailed the man. 'Please, make them hurry! I need an ambulance.'

'Forget the ambulance! And certainly forget cutting the cord! All you need to do is help her get the baby out,' I instructed. 'Now, do as I say! Are you ready?'

All the maternity instructions are built into the AMPDS software, which is fortunate as BBAs are fairly rare and we don't get much practice! I brought up the screen and skipped the bit about getting towels and cushions and blankets – there was no time for that.

'With each contraction place the palm of your hand against the baby's head,' I read. 'As the baby delivers, support its head and shoulders. Remember, it will be slippery – do not drop it!'

The father relayed these instructions to the patient's mother (the baby's grandmother) who was also in the room.

'Where is she supposed to put her hand again?'

'Against the baby's head. I mean, against that thing . . .'

The mother-to-be screamed in the background.

'Oh my God!' said the father. 'I think she's in serious trouble! I think she's dying! She's in so much pain, and there's blood, and this white stuff, and water and it's all gone like, oh my God! HELP! Send the ambulance!'

It took me a good couple of minutes to persuade him that nothing was actually going wrong and that this was all normal. With the next contraction he got it together, and encouraged the mother to 'Puuuush!' and take deep breaths and do all those things that happen when people give birth on TV. After this contraction the whole of the head was out.

'Oh my God!' said the father. 'It's the baby's head!' I think that, up until this point, he had seen the protrusions from his girlfriend's vagina as something totally alien and had forgotten the fact that she was having a baby at all. I was just relieved that it hadn't been a foot – breech births are far more dangerous and really need to be dealt with in hospital.

A slight problem then occurred in that, after three more contractions, no more of the baby emerged. It was time to change tack.

'Get the mother sitting on a cushion,' I told him, 'and tell her to grab her legs and pull them over her shoulders. Then, with the next contraction, tell her to push really hard.'

The mother did as she was told. Childbirth is indeed not a dignified process. There was an ear-splitting scream, and then a lot of crying. It was hard to pick out the sound of the baby crying, because the father was crying, the mother was crying, and so was the grandmother. I was the only person not crying.

'Is the baby breathing?' I asked, crossing my fingers.

'Yes, it's crying!' said the father. There was then a short break while everyone was sighing and gasping and saying things such as 'Oh my God' and 'I can't believe it'.

'Right,' I said. 'Clean the baby's mouth and nose, wrap it up and give it to the mother. What have you got, a boy or a girl?'

There was a pause while he had a look. Then he came back to the phone. 'Um, I can't tell!'

It is kind of worrying that someone who can make a baby doesn't know the fundamentals of reproductive anatomy!

The ambulance arrived shortly after that – the whole thing had happened in less than five minutes. Mother and baby were well, and were taken to hospital to be checked over. The sex of the baby remains a mystery.

# Overdose

25 February 2006

Three calls after my fourth Born Before Arrival, I was still sitting there with a grin on my face. It's not often we get a happy call in Ambulance Control – usually the best we can hope for is improving a bad situation – so when something good happens, we like to savour the moment.

My bubble was, however, quickly broken.

'It's my flatmate,' said a male voice with a thick foreign accent. 'I think he's overdosed ...'

Because of his accent it took almost a minute to get the address correctly, with him spelling out every word. C for Charlie, H for Heroin ... Eventually I had the address correct and moved on to the questioning.

'How old is he?'

'Twenty-eight.'

'Is he conscious?'

'No ...'

Uh oh! 'Is he breathing?'

'Um ... no, I don't think he is ...'

Aargh!

I can't quite describe the sinking feeling you get when you have been struggling to get an address from a caller and you realize that the delay may have cost the patient his life. If only I understood foreign accents better, if only callers could brush up on their English ... But of course, there is no point in 'if only's at a time like this.

Since the caller wasn't entirely sure that his flatmate wasn't breathing, it was time to crank up the 'respiration timer'. As I've mentioned before, it is very hard to get some callers to concentrate long enough to use it correctly, but I didn't have any problems with this one. In fact, he was eerily calm and compliant. I suspect he had been taking some of whatever his flatmate had (although he later informed me that he didn't know what kind of drug it was and had just stumbled across him in this state). From timing the breaths it seemed that they were indeed agonal, so I pressed on with resuscitation. Much to my relief the language barrier didn't stop the caller understanding the instructions. We do have an interpreter service, but trying to use it for complicated instructions usually results in chaos, calamity and – ultimately – death.

The phone was right by the patient, so I could hear the full gamut of gruesome sound effects.

*Puff!* *Hisssss* *Puff!* *Hisssssssssss*

*Clunk* *Clunk* *Clunk* *Clunk* *Clunk* *Clunk* *Clunk* *Clunk*

*Clunk* *Clunk* *Clunk* *Clunk* *Clunk* *Clunk* *Clunk*

*Bluuuuuurgh!* *Wipe*

*Puff!* *Hisssss* *Puff!* *Hisssssssssss*

When callers are very calm like this one in the face of a 'suspended' patient, I am often overcome with a sense of paranoia that the patient isn't really suspended and that they have misunderstood me, resulting in them leaping up and down on and breaking the ribs of a perfectly healthy patient. This was particularly strong in this case because the patient was so young and, although the caller's English seemed perfect (except for his accent), maybe he thought I had said something else entirely. Still, I told myself that I had checked several times and that it was much better to break the ribs of a live patient than ignore a dying one.

The ambulance arrived and I proceeded to continually check the log to see what happened next. Eventually, after forty long minutes, the ambulance set off to the nearest hospital on blue lights. The patient was indeed suspended, and had stayed that way despite the ambulance crew zapping him with the defibrillator and doing whatever else it is ambulance crews do to prevent suspended patients turning into corpses. Although they were taking him into hospital, his chances were slim, and we later heard that he had been pronounced dead in A&E.

So, as the family two miles down the road were cradling their new baby and waiting for the midwife to come and determine its sex once and for all, this young man was saying goodbye to the world for ever. He was my age. What a tragic waste of a life.

# No Need to Panic?

So there I was, minding my own business, when the Area Controller from the north-east desk came along and waved an ambulance call receipt in front of my nose.

'Remember this one, Suzi?'

I racked my brains. A call I'd taken around an hour ago. 24 Fortress Road, N23. Seventeen-year-old female having a panic attack. Bells started ringing somewhere in the back of my mind. Oh yes, I remembered it now.

'Do you remember anything out of the ordinary about it?' asked the Area Controller.

'Um,' I said, scratching my head. 'Well, the caller was a bit of an idiot, but nothing unusual, no.'

The call had gone something like this.

Me: ...
Caller: YES! RIGHT! WE NEED AN AMBULANCE HERE NOW!

Me: WHAT'S –
Caller: SHE'S HAVING ONE OF HER ATTACKS!
Patient in background: AARGH, OOH, HELP ME!

Me: WHAT KIND OF ATTACK?
Caller: IT'S A PANIC ATTACK.

Me: AND WHAT'S THE ADDRESS?
Caller: 24 FORTRESS ROAD, N23. LOOK, MAN, NEVER MIND ALL THIS, JUST GET HERE QUICK!
Patient in background: I'M DYING, I'M DYING!

**Me:** OKAY, I NEED TO ASK YOU A FEW QUESTIONS, BUT –
**Caller:** I AIN'T GOT TIME! JUST SEND THE AMBULANCE!

**Me:** IF YOU COULD LET ME FINISH ... I WAS GOING TO SAY THAT
   I NEED TO ASK YOU QUESTIONS, HELP WILL BE ARRANGED WHILE
   I'M TALKING TO YOU.
**Caller:** SHE'S DYING, SHE'S DYING.

**Me:** PLEASE TRY TO CALM DOWN. SHE'S HAVING A PANIC ATTACK,
   SHE ISN'T DYING.

These were the words that would come back to haunt me.

The rest of the call proceeded in much the same manner. I managed to extract the relevant information: she was seventeen, conscious and breathing, and the call was categorized as red because the patient was hyperventilating, in other words, not breathing normally. This is usually the way with panic attacks and I have always thought it was a bit of a waste of an ambulance, because there is nothing an ambulance crew can do to help other than be nice and calm the patient down, which is something anyone can do. Still, off it went and I gave it no further thought. Until ...

'So, go on ...' I asked the Area Controller. 'What was strange about it?'

'We've just blued in a 55-year-old female from that address,' the Area Controller explained. 'Suspended.' ('Blued in' refers to the process of taking a critically ill patient to hospital on blue lights and pre-alerting the hospital.)

'Oh my God!' I exclaimed, clapping a hand over my mouth. 'I've killed her!'

'I'm sure it's not your fault,' said the Area Controller. 'What did they say on the phone?'

I told him, and he looked as confused as I felt.

I started to panic. The call had been a red, but in my head I had thought it should have been a green. Had I missed something the caller said that could have alerted me to how serious the situation was? If I'd stayed on the phone, could I have given life-saving instructions? The caller had told me the patient was dying, and I'd thought he was being silly, but he was right.

I knew that if I'd done something wrong, I'd be called to the Coroner's Court and the tape would be played back in front of everyone. I'd have to justify to this poor woman's family why I had hung up and left her to die. I racked my brains, trying to remember the conversation. Was it my fault? I spent an anxious hour watching the movements of the ambulance that had conveyed the patient to hospital, and as soon as they arrived back on station, I gave them a call.

'You know that suspended you just did ...' I ventured.

'Oh God, what now?' said the paramedic, alarmed.

'No, nothing!' I said. 'I took the call and I just wondered how on earth a 17-year-old having a panic attack turned into a 55-year-old suspended?'

'God knows!' he said. 'It was a madhouse in there, and we came in to find her lying in the hallway, looking pretty dead, so we didn't stop to ask questions. But there were definitely no panicking seventeen-year-olds there. There was just her and a man, they'd both been on the drink, and there was evidence of drug taking too, so I think that's what did it. Her lungs were full of fluid – even with the suction we couldn't get anywhere.'

'I'm really worried that I messed up the call,' I told him.

'I don't think it's your fault – he wasn't on this planet!' he said. 'We've left him with the police.'

'How is the patient?' I ventured.

'Dead,' said the paramedic solemnly.

After I'd finished on the phone, Management came over to me.

'Suzi, we heard what happened and we've been to listen to the tape ...' he began.

I gulped.

'It was exactly as you remembered – he said the patient was seventeen and having a panic attack. There was no way you could have known.'

Despite the unfavourable outcome for the patient, I felt incredibly relieved. It's obvious there was a lot more to this call than met the eye, and nothing that could have been guessed from the call.

I tell you what, though – that's the last time I tell a patient that they're not dying.

# Banana Man

10 March 2006

I will never understand why some people think it is funny or clever to hoax call the emergency services. Hoax calls cost lives. While ambulance crews drive round in circles trying to find patients that don't exist and accidents that never happened, and Control staff waste hours on the phone trying to determine the location of fictitious incidents, other, genuine patients are put in danger.

The vast majority of hoaxes come from children, most of whom, I hope, get a stern talking-to from their parents when the ambulance turns up (children tend not to realize that we can trace any landline call, and the owner of any registered mobile!), and then they never do it again. There are also a fair few hoax calls from older teenagers, who, I'm guessing, are doing it for a dare. This type of hoax is pretty easy to spot – the call is usually blurted out in a rehearsed manner and involves 'someone' plus a medical diagnosis, rather than the more usual description of what has happened. ('Someone's broken their leg!' as opposed to 'My brother fell down the stairs and his leg hurts!') The caller usually hangs up on further questioning, without giving an address. If they do give an address, it's usually a main road. I can't ever remember taking a hoax call and not realizing it was a hoax at the time, which makes it all the more frustrating because, unless we've already been to the address that day, we have to treat every single call as if it were genuine.

Somewhat more sinister are the regular hoaxers. We've had a few of these over the years. Some have been prosecuted, but some we never find. If a caller uses an unregistered mobile or a payphone to call, it's pretty much impossible to trace them. There was one young woman who called us every night for months, giving an address near her own every time. When she was eventually traced, she was found to be mentally ill and to have an obsession with ambulances. Her bedroom wall was covered with pictures of them and she was calling 999 just so she could see one outside. There was also a spate of hoaxes to one address, which were believed to be coming from the ex-partner of the person who lived there. They always gave outlandish reasons such as a house on fire or a plane crash, and on one occasion, 'My wife has cut my testicles off and cooked them in the oven.'

This week, we've been utterly inundated with calls from possibly the most annoying hoaxer ever. He's been calling us for a couple of months now, but this week the call rate has gone through the roof. I'd say he is calling a couple of hundred times a day. Each call taker will end up speaking to him around ten times per shift. Of course, we've had his mobile cut off – we do this by sending a report to the mobile phone provider – but he just goes out and buys a new one, and he's back again. He gives his address as 10 Bethnal Green Road, E1. He says it like this: 'Ten, Bethnal Green Ro-ho-ad! Number Te-hen!' This address doesn't actually exist – Bethnal Green Road runs from E1 to E2, and if there was a number 10, which there isn't, it would be in E2. When you put the address into the computer, it tries to work out where it would be, and as a result directs the ambulance crews to a Woolworth's.

This guy thinks he is hilarious. He loves to give his diagnosis as 'itchy penis' and I think this is just because he is amused by the word 'penis'. Sometimes he will just call up and laugh and say that he needs an ambulance because he or his girlfriend (surely a moron like this cannot possibly have a girlfriend?) cannot stop laughing. Sometimes he will just sing his 'address' at us and laugh hysterically. He knows that we cannot hang up on someone if they say they need an ambulance, so he will always maintain that he needs an ambulance, despite rarely giving a coherent reason. Lately he has given up on giving any medical reasons for needing us whatsoever – instead he will alternately offer the call taker a banana, or request that a banana is brought to him. According to one rather exasperated emergency operator

I spoke to, when asked 'Emergency, which service? Police, fire or ambulance?' he replied 'Greengrocer'.

If I didn't think it would lose me my job, I would quite happily give Banana Man's phone number to every EMD in the room and instruct them to call him, preferably at three in the morning, and offer him random items of fruit and veg and see how *he* likes it.

# I Thought it Would Make Them Come Quicker

## 14 March 2006

Sometimes when the call comes in, the level of background noise is such that I actually recoil and have to move my headphone away from my ear slightly. This was one of those calls. What sounded like fifteen people were shouting and screaming.

'What's the problem?' I asked.

'Ambulance!' said a foreign male.

'What's the problem?' I asked.

'It's an emergency!' screamed a hysterical woman.

'What's the problem?' I asked.

'Get 'ere quick!' bellowed a gruff-sounding man.

'What's the problem?' I asked.

'Ambulance, naaaaaah!' said a squeaky teenager.

I tried a difference tack.

'What's the address of the emergency?'

'Shot!' said yet another voice. 'He's been shot!'

'What's the address of the emergency?' I asked, feeling nervous and excited at the same time – I've never taken a call about a shooting before.

'Sorry, what was that?' said a reasonably sensible-sounding young man.

'Okay, okay, *please*, don't give the phone to anyone else. What's the address?'

'It's a chicken shop ... Bernard's Fried Chicken in Dicey Broadway in Peckham ... I just saw all these people screaming and panicking, so I came over to see what was going on ... hey, everyone, what *is* going on?'

'Be careful!' I ordered. 'Someone's been shot. Don't go in there unless you're sure it's safe. Get someone to come out and give you some information, if you can?'

It took another couple of minutes before anyone came out of the shop to talk to the man, and getting information out of him was not easy when they did.

'How many people have been hurt?'

'One – a little boy, he's about one ...'

'Oh my God,' I thought, 'they've shot a baby!'

'And the person who shot him? Are they still near by?'

'Shot?' said the man from the shop. 'He ain't been shot!'

'But someone said there'd been a shooting!' I protested.

'Oh, naaah,' said the man, without a hint of shame. 'He just said that so you'd get down here quick, like.'

'So, what is wrong?' I asked.

'Well, the baby, it wasn't breathing, like, but now it is, right ...' (I suspect the baby had had a fit – otherwise people don't usually stop and start breathing randomly, just like that.)

By this point several police cars, an ambulance and a duty officer were all on their way to a meet-up point near by in order to arrive on the scene en masse. Ambulances don't go into crime scenes until they are given police clearance to do so. I had to get a message to the dispatch desk pronto that there was no shooting and that everyone could be stood down, except the ambulance, which needed to get to the sick baby sharpish.

I would have given the caller a lecture about how lying to the emergency services wastes everyone's time and, in this case, would actually have caused a delay in reaching the baby, had the lie not been uncovered. But I was too busy banging my head on the desk with exasperation.

# Help the Aged

## 26 March 2006

It's not uncommon for calls to make a dent in my faith in humanity. Usually, however, that dent is made by the behaviour of the caller, rather than the nature of the emergency itself.

It was my first call of the shift, just before 7 a.m. Like most calls this time of day, it was from a distressed-sounding elderly lady.

'Help me!' she squealed. 'There's blood everywhere!'

The usual cause of a call like this is piles, closely followed by falls and other minor injuries. Old people have papery skin and a lot of them are on blood thinners, so they often generate a lot of blood.

'Okay, we can get you some help,' I said in my best reassuring voice. 'Can you tell me what's happened?'

'There was someone here,' said the little old lady. 'He came in through the window!'

'You've had a break-in?' I said, realizing that this was not a routine call after all. 'Did the burglar attack you?'

'Yes!' said the old lady in a trembling voice. 'Oh, please come, please help me! I'm ninety-three!'

'Of course, we'll come straight away,' I told her (and yes, I know I'm not supposed to say that, but I don't think I'm going to get sacked for it). 'Is the man who did this still there?'

'I don't know!' said the lady.

What would I have told her to do if he was – run away? She was ninety-three, she wouldn't have got very far. Fortunately, the carer turned up at that precise moment. I could hear her in the background.

'Mrs Bell? Mrs Bell! What on earth has happened? The front

door was open and there's ... oh my goodness, what has happened to you? Who are you talking to?'

The carer came to the phone and I explained who I was and that the police and ambulance were coming. I was concerned, though, that the intruder might still be around, so after triaging the call I stayed on the line with the carer, instructing her not to leave the room until the police arrived. Fortunately, they were on the scene within a few minutes, closely followed by the ambulance.

This must have been one of the most horrible calls I have taken, simply because I cannot imagine what would motivate someone to attack a 93-year-old woman. I can see the motivation behind most crimes — stealing for financial gain, assault as revenge — but what gain is there in this? She was hardly going to prevent them from burgling the house at her age, so it couldn't be considered a display of bravado. Someone of ninety-three should be living out their days in peace and quiet and not have their last memories polluted with such ugly violence.

I hope whoever did this gets caught, and I hope they lie awake at night haunted by their own cowardly act of bullying.

# I Despair ...

Someone actually called for an ambulance for an ingrowing toe-nail last night ...

No, they didn't get one.

# Last Breath

One call reminded me of just how close to incidents we really do get as call takers. It was a call from an elderly lady who was a carer for her even more elderly friend. Her friend had suddenly started vomiting a lot of bright red blood which, as you can imagine, is not a good sign. The call came out as a red call, which would usually have meant an ambulance in under eight minutes. But, unfortunately, they lived in one of those pesky 'rural' places that is at least eight minutes' drive on blue lights from the nearest ambulance station. (Within the London Ambulance catchment area you are never more than about fifteen minutes' drive from your nearest ambulance station. In, say, Yorkshire plenty of people are forty-five minutes or more from the nearest ambulance station – and the poor call takers have to stay on the line all that time, and the callers *still* expect the ambulance to be there in five seconds flat! It must be even worse for Americans and Australians . . .) The nearest ambulance and FRU were sent. They weren't very near at all – five miles and seven miles away respectively.

While I was asking the triage questions, I could hear the patient groaning and vomiting in the background. She sounded in a bad way and I prayed the traffic would be on our side and that the FRU would get there more quickly than the computer's estimate of ten minutes. Of course, there is one thing worse than a patient sounding really ill in the background, and that's a patient who you can't hear at all. And that's precisely what happened next. Just as I was telling the caller to put her dogs away and open the door, everything went quiet.

'Doris? Doris! She's gone unconscious! Help!'

My poor caller, who up until this point had sounded calm – as if she had been calling ambulances for Doris on a regular basis – totally panicked. After having the usual 'Where's the ambulance/hurry up/why's it taking so long?' conversation, I tried to move on to the instructions for an unconscious person. But it was no good. Doris, who was in her late eighties, had collapsed in an armchair with her head lolling to one side. Joan, the caller, sounded a little younger, but not much, and was totally unable to lift her unconscious friend from the chair to the floor. Their nearest neighbour was a few minutes' walk away and Joan told me she couldn't walk very fast, so there was no point going for help. It's always a difficult judgement to make as to whether you should encourage or even pressurize a caller into moving a patient when they feel unable to do so. On the one hand, it might only be the fear of making things worse that is stopping them (Joan started off by saying she couldn't put Doris on the floor, Doris had a bad hip, it could hurt her ... but alive with a broken hip is better than dead without ...), and on the other hand, they really might be physically incapable and could even injure themselves trying, and then we'd end up with two patients instead of one! So I didn't push Joan any further, and instead concentrated on getting her to try to open Doris's airway while she was still in the armchair, to clean the blood away from her mouth, talk to her and generally make her comfortable.

I decided to use the 'breath timer' gadget on the computer. Normally we use this for a patient with abnormal breathing, to determine whether they are going into cardiac arrest and whether CPR needs to be started. On this occasion I already knew that CPR wouldn't be possible, but I thought I would do it anyway – partly to give Joan a 'job' to make her feel she was doing something, and partly so that I could convey this information to the FRU and ambulance in order to better prepare them if she did stop breathing.

The first time I used the gadget, Doris's breathing was a nice, regular pattern. A little slow, but acceptable. Joan reassured Doris that she was going to be fine. Doris was silent.

The second time I did it, Doris's breathing had slowed down a lot. The gadget told me this was possibly an agonal pattern and to start CPR or recheck. I rechecked. This time, Doris's breathing was irregular, alternating between shallow and rattling gasps with long gaps in between. I had no doubt that she was arresting.

Just as I was changing the 'breathing?' answer from 'yes' to 'agonal' on the ticket, the FRU burst through the door. I heard him talk to Joan briefly and look at Doris before picking up and speaking to me. I already guessed what he was going to say.

'She's suspended, can you ask for a second vehicle, please? Thanks.'

And then they were gone. The dispatch desk got the second vehicle there and Doris was blued into hospital in cardiac arrest, but she didn't make it.

You could spend a lot of time worrying about a call like this and how it could have been done differently. If Doris and Joan had lived closer to town, or if we'd had an ambulance on standby in their village, would we have reached them more quickly? And would that have made any difference? If I'd sent Joan to fetch the neighbour, or been a bit pushier with her, would CPR have been started earlier and saved Doris's life? Or would she have died alone while Joan was fetching the neighbour? Would Joan have hurt her back and been unable to comfort Doris as she took her dying breaths? I'll never know, but I hope I did the right thing.

Sometimes making someone's death more comfortable is better than trying to save their life.

# Prize for Stupidity

15 April 2006

Somewhere in the depths of north London a young man fell over and injured his leg. He thought it might be broken. He hobbled to the telephone and dialled the number of his local taxi firm. Yes, that's a real taxi, not one of our Big White ones. He then limped outside to wait for the taxi. Ten minutes later it arrived, and he eased himself into the back seat.

'Where to?' asked the cab driver, starting the engine and pulling off.

'North Middlesex Hospital, please,' said the man. 'The A&E department. I think I've broken my leg!'

'Oh my God!' said the taxi driver. 'You can't be getting in a taxi with a broken leg. Hold on a minute!'

He drove to the firm's headquarters and used their phone to dial 999, explaining that he had a man with a broken leg in his taxi asking to be taken to the hospital. He got through to me.

'Erm,' I said, hating to state the bleeding obvious. 'He's got a broken leg, and he's in your taxi asking to be taken to the hospital. Why don't you take him there? If we send an ambulance, we're just going to have to take him out of the taxi, which will mean moving him around, and if someone has a broken bone you're supposed to move them as little as possible.'

'Look, mate,' said the taxi driver gruffly, 'he's got a broken leg, he's ENTITLED to an ambulance! Stop trying to get out of sending him one!'

'I'm quite happy to send an ambulance,' I said (this was a lie), 'it's just that if a patient with a broken leg is in a car, it makes more sense and is better for the patient to drive him straight to the hospital.'

'Right!' said the taxi driver, and left the phone.

In the background I could hear muffled voices and a young man cursing in pain. It sounded rather like he was being dragged out of the back of the taxi.

The taxi driver returned. 'We've got him out!' he said triumphantly. 'Now send us an ambulance!'

*Click*

# How Not to Succeed in Sales

17 April 2006

**Me:** EMERGENCY AMBULANCE, WHAT IS THE ADDRESS OF THE EMERGENCY?

**Caller:** GOOD MORNING. THIS IS MR GERALD BROWNING, CALLING FROM BROWNING EMERGENCY SYSTEMS.

**Me:** OKAY, AND WHAT IS THE ADDRESS OF THE EMERGENCY, PLEASE?

**Caller:** NO, *I* DON'T HAVE AN EMERGENCY. I'M RINGING TO TELL YOU ABOUT OUR NEW PRODUCT, THE BROWNING EMERGENCY VACU-LIFT. PERHAPS I COULD FAX YOU ACROSS SOME BROCHURES?

**Me:** YOU'RE RINGING 999 TO TRY AND SELL ME SOME AMBULANCE EQUIPMENT?

**Caller:** YES ... SORRY, THIS IS THE AMBULANCE SERVICE, ISN'T IT?

**Me:** YOU'RE BLOCKING AN EMERGENCY LINE AND POTENTIALLY ENDANGERING LIVES TO SELL US YOUR PRODUCT. I HARDLY THINK WE ARE GOING TO BE INTERESTED IN BUYING ANYTHING WITH SUCH A LACK OF AWARENESS OF EMERGENCY SYSTEMS. I'M GOING TO HANG UP NOW. GOODBYE, MR BROWNING.

# The Interrupter

One of the most irritating events in the world for us call takers (and believe me, there are a lot of events that irritate us) is the phenomenon of the Interrupter. Picture this: some kind of emergency is going on, and a helpful sensible person has called 999. You've explained to them that someone will arrange help while you ask a few questions, and they're calmly giving you the information you need.

Now enter the Interrupter. The Interrupter will invariably wrestle the phone from the original caller and, without giving you a chance to get a word in edgeways, will pompously bellow at you: 'High Street! Outside Tesco! We need an ambulance here now. You need to get here fast! This is an emergency!' A really, really unhelpful statement, since you got the address (including which High Street and where Tesco is) two minutes ago, you know they need an ambulance because you work for the Ambulance Service and they wouldn't be calling you otherwise, you figured it was indeed an emergency when the first caller told you a guy had been hit by a bus and, strangely enough, ambulances tend to get to places fast by virtue of the fact that they drive through red lights, on the wrong side of the road, etc. Do they think that you are going to send a 'slow ambulance' unless they request a fast one? If you are lucky, they will follow this up with a lecture about how you are incompetent, wasting time, asking stupid questions, etc., and how they are going to put in a formal complaint about you. After that they invariably hang up, which in a way is a good thing, because it prevents us being able to answer back in a knee-jerk way that really would give them something to complain about.

Anyway, a prime example of the Interrupter occurred the other day. It was the early hours of the morning and some kind of drama had occurred, resulting in a 32-year-old man being stabbed. I could tell straight away it was serious. The girlfriend, who made the call, was absolutely hysterical at first (as you would be), and just kept shouting 'He's been stabbed!', the name of the road, 'Help me!' and 'Oh my God, there's blood everywhere!' Fortunately, she'd called from a landline, so I cheated and grabbed the full address from that. The police were informed and an ambulance immediately dispatched, giving me a bit of leeway in deciding what to do next. After establishing that the attacker had scarpered, I got the caller and her female friend to try and bring the bleeding under control with an assortment of cloths and tea towels. The friend did this, while the girlfriend stayed on the phone. She calmed down a little once this had been done, and I was able to go through the rest of the questions. Despite being terrified and still crying her eyes out, she managed to answer me (between 'aargh's and 'oh God, help, he's dying's). Her boyfriend was indeed in a bad way, unconscious with multiple deep stab wounds to the chest and back. He'd been breathing at the start of the call, but I wasn't sure this would last long, so I asked if he was still breathing now.

'Erm,' she said, 'I don't know ... I think he just took a breath ... he's not breathing now ... aargh! Help! Wait, he took a breath ...'

It sounded like agonal breathing. I knew it was time to get ready for CPR. But the girlfriend was upset enough as it was – would she be together enough to do it?

At that point I heard a relatively calm voice in the background telling the caller to give her the phone. I guessed this belonged to a neighbour and felt relieved – she would be detached enough to either do CPR herself, or take control of the situation and get one of the others doing it right. I happily let Distraught But Helpful Girlfriend give her the phone.

You've guessed it – the neighbour was the Interrupter.

'Look,' she said crossly, 'we've already called an ambulance – and the police as well! Just get here!'

*Click*

Disaster.

I called back twice, leaving messages asking them to call back straight away, but no one answered and no one called back. The FRU was on the scene a few minutes later, and the patient was in respiratory arrest. By the time he was blued into hospital, the patient had been in asystole ('flatline' – in other words, very little hope) for twenty minutes. He was pronounced dead in hospital.

From the crew's reports, it seemed very unlikely that the patient would have survived, even with immediate CPR – 'skewered' was the word they used to describe him. Nonetheless, in situations like these, we always like to feel that we did everything we could for the patient and gave him every possible chance. Thanks to the Interrupter, that wasn't possible in this case.

# Passing On the Bad Habits

26 April 2006

I have been given a call-taking trainee to teach my bad habits to! The first I heard about it was approximately ten minutes before she arrived, when a member of Management appeared, thrust a pair of trainee epaulettes in my direction and barked, 'These are for your trainee!'

I didn't even have time to ask, 'What trainee?' before Management had gone away again.

My trainee is called Angela and she is a few years older than me. She used to be an auxiliary nurse. She is actually very good at the job already – she has a calm and reassuring manner, and I've even picked some tips up from her. I've said before that the finer points of call taking aren't something you can teach and, listening to Angela, I feel that's truer than ever. It's a relief to know she has 'got it' because I'd feel so awkward trying to teach someone while knowing they are never going to fit in here.

There was no gradual induction to call taking for Angela – we had a BBA (my fifth) on the first morning, and later on that day Angela's first suspended (an elderly man who'd seemingly had a heart attack). Afterwards I asked Angela if she wanted to take a stress break in case she was traumatized from hearing someone die. She replied in the negative – apparently when she was an auxiliary nurse, patients died in front of her all the time and it's like water off a duck's back to her now! Well, that told me.

# Driving Lessons

It's my birthday! I am twenty-nine years old. Alan bought me some new bandages for my first-aid kit. It was very thoughtful of him. My mother's gift was even better – she has paid for me to have ten hours' worth of driving lessons. If they all go well, I'll do my driving test at the end and then I'll think seriously about applying for the next Student Paramedic Course.

Driving is hard work. After two hours' tuition I can now turn left *and* right *and* change gears. The problems only start when I try to combine the three. I also have difficulty getting the car to go in the direction I intend it to and getting it to stop in the right place without giving myself whiplash. I think it is safe to say that driving is not something I am naturally skilled at. I usually pick things up quite quickly and tell myself I can do anything if I set my mind to it, but this is proving to be an uphill struggle.

I have a week's annual leave to celebrate my birthday. Alan and I are going to Brighton for a few days. Back to work on 10 May.

# Banana Man Relocates

10 May 2006

Having worked out that we are no longer sending ambulances to the address that might just be a Woolworth's in the East End, our obsessive hoaxer has now taken to telling us he is at Gatwick Airport. Sitting on the runway. Suffering from an itchy penis. Offering us bananas. I must have spoken to him twenty times last night.

I swear that if I ever come across this individual, I will do something with a banana that necessitates a genuine phone call to the emergency services.

# Thank You

12 May 2006

Today Angela stayed on the phone giving instructions to the daughter of an unconscious diabetic lady for ten minutes until the ambulance arrived. Afterwards the crew rang to pass on the daughter's thanks! She described Angela as 'really calm and professional'. Angela was very pleased. So was I – it's not often we get thanked. I can count on the fingers of one hand the number of times I've had similar messages, so for Angela to get one this early in her career will do her self-esteem the world of good and hopefully convince her to stay in the job long term.

# Taking Out the Rubbish

17 May 2006

Angela took a call on her shift from a careline. Carelines are a service for elderly/disabled people who live alone. They have a pendant around their neck that they press if they need help and can't make it to the phone themselves. They then talk via the careline alarm unit and explain to the operator what the problem is, and the careline call us and either give us instructions on how to get in or send someone round with a key.

'What's the problem?' asked Angela.

'Mrs White was taking the rubbish out when she slipped and somehow fell bottom first into the dustbin! She says she's fine, she's not hurt, but she just can't get out!'

I couldn't help it. I giggled. I had to move the headset away from my mouth in case the careline heard me. The more I tried not to laugh, the more I wanted to. It wasn't funny really, but it was just the thought of an old lady stuck in a dustbin with her arms and legs sticking out! Luckily Angela was very professional and her voice didn't waver a jot as she took the details.

# More Driving Lessons

19 May 2006

Today was my fifth and final driving lesson from the set my mother paid for. My driving instructor finished up with a mock test and made a list of all the things on which I would have failed. They are as follows.

- Turning right in a small gap in the traffic. ('You can't go in there! What if that other car was breaking the speed limit?')

- *Not* turning right in a small gap in the traffic. ('What are you waiting for? Go! No, too late!')

- Driving too close to parked cars when overtaking them.

- Driving *too far out* from parked cars when overtaking them. ('But you said I was too close last time!' 'Yes, but this time there is a lamppost with an orange light, an "r" in the month and a bus lane on Sundays, so you should drive closer.')

- Driving at 35 mph in a 30 mph zone. (Even though all the other cars were doing at least 40 mph, and were honking their horns at me reprovingly and overtaking with a whoosh.)

- Not looking in every single mirror before speeding up, slowing down or breathing.

- Driving at 90 mph, on the wrong side of the road, through red traffic lights without blue flashing lights on top of the car.

On the whole I'm really not sure if I want to continue with my lessons. When I look at the effortless way Steve cut through the traffic in a five-ton ambulance and consider that I can't even drive a lousy Corsa in a straight line without endangering the public, I think that maybe my future is within the control room for ever. Also, staying in the control room means I will never have to deal with vomit in real life (unless Alan gets too drunk at a party).

# An Odd Request

Management have signed Angela off, so she is now taking calls on her own. I felt unreasonably sad that she didn't need me any more. It was like waving your child off for her first day at school. I spent the rest of the day solo call taking once more and feeling a trifle lonely. Still, now I don't have a trainee to look after Management have agreed to let me go on another observation shift with Steve and Barry. It's been arranged for the beginning of July, which is a convenient point in the rota.

The most 'interesting' call today came around lunchtime, from an extremely drunk-sounding male. He didn't want an ambulance, he told me, but he had no credit on his phone and didn't know what else to do. I expected he was going to ask me to contact his GP or social worker as people sometimes do, but no.

'I hear Richard Branson is making a space rocket,' he told me. 'And I need to tell him how to do it.'

I was, for once, lost for words.

'Um,' I said. 'We don't have any dealings with Richard Branson. Are you sure you don't need an ambulance?'

'I told you I didn't!' said the man (as if I was the one saying the stupid things). 'Richard Branson is sending a rocket into space, and he needs my help.'

'Well, this is an ambulance service,' I said. 'What makes you think we have anything to do with Richard Branson?'

'You're all British, aren't you?' said the man, and promptly hung up.

When I got home, I Googled 'Richard Branson space rocket' and found that Richard Branson *is* actually sending a rocket into space. This was news to me. You learn something new every day in this job …

# Alan Has an Accident

23 May 2006

It seems that I just can't keep away from ambulances – even on my day off.

On Saturday night Alan and I went to our friend Maria's house-warming party, deep in the depths of west London. It was a very decadent party, with an outdoor jacuzzi, a chocolate fountain and, er, a Eurovision sweepstake. About 2 a.m. I suddenly started to feel rather tired and needed to lie down. This may well have had something to do with the four pints of beer, bottle of wine, glass of congealed toffee/chocolate/cherry cocktail and fifty-nine vodka jellies I had consumed.

An hour or so later I was awakened by Maria, bellowing: 'SUZI, SUZI! ALAN HAS CUT HIS ARM! QUICK! QUICK!'

I'd like to say I was a dutiful girlfriend and rushed to his aid, but in fact I muttered something about plasters and pulled the duvet over my head. Maria was opening and shutting her mouth and there was noise coming out, but it didn't seem to make much sense, and I hoped she would go away as each word was like a ten-ton weight dropping on my head.

'Call an ambulance! I think it's an arterial bleed!' shouted someone else, and this finally jolted me into awakeness. 'Ambulance' is obviously the magic word you need to get my attention. I staggered into the living room, and there were several thousand people running around, some of them in bikinis, flapping their arms and throwing tea towels around the room. In the middle of the chaos, lying in a pool of blood, was Alan.

'Look!' he said, raising the affected limb to show everyone. 'Blood everywhere! I've practically cut it off!'

As he waved the arm, the tea towel Maria's flatmate was diligently holding against the wound slipped, and a torrent of blood spurted out and caught him in the face. I decided to pretend this was all one big training exercise and did all the lying-down, applying-pressure, raising-the-injured limb, etc. stuff while Maria called the ambulance.

'My friend's here! She works in Control! Speak to her!' said Maria.

I cringed, took the phone and answered the questions of an unimpressed-sounding call taker.

'So what exactly happened?' I finally asked. It seemed Alan had been heading for the jacuzzi in the garden and feeling his way along a wall. The wall had actually been a garden shed. With a window in it. Alan had leant on the window, it had given way and cut his arm to shreds.

It was 3 a.m. on a Saturday night/Sunday morning, which I knew was a very busy time, and therefore maybe we'd be in for a long wait, so I was very impressed that an FRU turned up after fifteen minutes. We ushered him in and all pretended to be sober, in the manner of fifteen-year-olds caught drinking by our parents. The FRU suspected a possible arterial bleed (although it didn't seem to be pumping quite the same way as the prisoner's face had when I was out on observation with Steve) and asked for an ambulance on the hurry-up.

Alan and I were bundled into the back of the ambulance and taken to the local hospital. The bleed, fortunately, was not arterial and Alan was sewn up and discharged. He wanted to go back to the party to show everyone his stitches, but I'd had enough and took him home.

All this drama reminded me that, despite the fact I am going off the idea of becoming a paramedic myself, I'm really looking forward to my observation shift out with Steve and Barry. It's still important for me to learn what the ambulance crews are actually doing – not to mention exciting!

# Abusive Callers Again

1 June 2006

For some reason the general public are in a bad mood today and I've been on the receiving end of some serious abuse. One man started calling me every name under the sun before I'd even had a chance to speak. In most jobs you would just hang up in the face of such language, but we're trained to react to callers' situations and not their attitude. I try to remember that it isn't personal and that the callers are only behaving like that because something awful is happening to them. Here – in my opinion – are the reasons why people are rude or abusive, and the types of rudeness that result.

1. *Personality of the caller.* You can't really do anything about this one except try not to make the situation worse. Some people are just plain rude. Sometimes it's a psychiatric problem, sometimes they just aren't very nice. For some reason, rude people are forever calling 999 – possibly because they have an exaggerated sense of entitlement, or because they like taking charge of situations.
2. *Panic.* Yes, panic is definitely a factor. Panicking people tend to lose all track of time (so they think the ambulance is taking ages, and they get angry) and have difficulty listening to what you are saying (causing frustration, because they don't understand what you are going on about) and it all comes out in a big rush of 'Just f★★★ing help me or I'll sue you!' Often by the end of the call they've calmed down and apologize or say thank you. Occasionally they even get the ambulance crews to ring Control with an apology for the call taker.
3. *Alcohol.* Definitely encourages rudeness, especially coupled with factor 1. Also encourages blathering and unhelpfulness. Drunken callers are definitely not my favourites.

4. *Not knowing the system.* Callers get frustrated because they have to answer lots of questions and because we don't know where 'the big road near Tesco in West London' is. They expect it to be like it is on TV. They think that if they are asked to do something to help the patient, we are trying to fob them off. They think that we should be telling them something more concrete at the end of the call ('We've dispatched an ambulance from Homerton and it will be with you in three minutes' rather than 'If his condition worsens, call back immediately for further instructions').

5. *Attitude of the call taker.* Some call takers seem to get more than their fair share of grief because of the way they react to rude callers. Getting cross is obviously a big no-no, but I think we've all had moments when we're exhausted and some horrible individual is shouting the odds at us, and we snap and answer back in a manner not depicted in any customer care manual. There are other ways in which we accidentally antagonize callers too. We constantly have to weigh up how the caller wants us to be, and then change our manner accordingly. Sometimes they feel we are too blasé and it comforts them if we pretend to be shocked at whatever they are reporting – but go too far and they will lose confidence in our ability to cope. Interrupt too little, and callers will waffle on, too much and they will get annoyed. Speak too fast and they will not understand us, too slowly and they will feel we have no sense of urgency. It's a constant balancing act and, given that we are not exactly getting callers when they are at their best, it's very easy to overbalance.

So now imagine a call where the caller is drunk, panicking, doesn't know the system, not a very nice person at the best of times, and doesn't think you're taking his situation very seriously. Yes, all five factors equal 'Call Taker Gets an Earful'. It's very rare to get a call from someone who is nice, calm and sober, knows the system, plus you respond correctly and manage not to upset them – thus almost every call leads to varying degrees of Earful.

Fortunately, we all have thick skins.

# Psychiatric Patients

6 June 2006

Psychiatric patients are some of my favourites, just behind deaf old people. I could sit and take calls from them all night.

I had the following conversation with a psychiatric patient yesterday.

Me: **EMERGENCY AMBULANCE, WHAT'S THE PROBLEM?**

Him: **(IN CALM AND FRIENDLY TONE.) I THINK I NEED TO GO TO A&E. I SELF-HARMED YESTERDAY.**

(At this point I am thinking, 'Yesterday? And you want an ambulance *now*? Timewaster!')

Me: **HOW OLD ARE YOU? ARE YOU FEELING VIOLENT? DO YOU HAVE ANY WEAPONS?**

Him: **(FAIRLY CHEERILY.) THIRTY-EIGHT. NO, I'M NOT VIOLENT. I JUST THINK I NEED TO SEE A PSYCHIATRIST AND GET MYSELF SORTED OUT. NOPE, NO WEAPONS HERE.**

Me: **AND WHEN YOU SELF-HARMED ... WHAT DID YOU DO?**

(I'm expecting him to say 'I cut my arms' at this point ...)

Him: **WELL, I TRIED TO CUT MY PENIS OFF! THAT'S NOT A GOOD THING, IS IT? SO I THINK I NEED TO GO TO HOSPITAL TO GET MY PENIS SORTED OUT. AND THEN SOME PSYCHIATRIC HELP TO MAKE SURE I DON'T DO IT AGAIN. OH YES! AND I TRIED TO BURN MY HOUSE DOWN WITH ME INSIDE IT. THEN I THOUGHT BETTER OF IT AND I MANAGED TO PUT THE FLAMES OUT! THAT WAS LUCKY, WASN'T IT? I DREAD TO THINK WHAT COULD HAVE HAPPENED!**

Me: OH! UM! ER! YES, I SEE. ER. ARE YOU BURNED? HOW IS YOUR
PENIS NOW?

Him: NO, I'M NOT BURNED. I MANAGED TO PUT IT OUT IN TIME. AND MY
PENIS JUST HAS SUPERFICIAL CUTS ON IT. IT'S HARDER TO CUT IT
OFF THAN YOU THINK, YOU KNOW.

(I have to say this isn't something that I have considered at great
length before, but is nice to know.)

The dispatch desk decided that our crew would wait for the police,
and a few minutes later we got a message from a rather shocked-
sounding police person: 'Ambulance ASAP please! Call as given!
Male is not very well!' We took him to the hospital and I hope he
managed to get himself into a good psych ward somewhere. I still
can't quite get my head around the way he was burning down his
house and chopping his bits off one minute, and then calmly and
almost cheerfully describing the events to me the next minute – as
if he were ringing about someone else!

# Choking Toddler

'This is Snowball Nursery in Southall,' cried the panicking nursery nurse, 'and we have a little boy choking on a rice cake!'

This was a proper case of complete obstruction choking – quite rare for us to come across as call takers, as most people realize that they have to do something straight away if someone is choking and that they don't have time to wait for an ambulance. Most of the choking calls we get are cases of partial obstruction, where all we do is encourage the patient to cough it up themselves and wait for the ambulance (backslapping in this case may encourage the obstruction to move and completely block the airway). The toddler was completely unable to breathe, turning blue and losing consciousness. The nursery staff had tried backslaps and the Heimlich manoeuvre without success.

I was glad I had the AMPDS software in front of me to prompt me, because this was a situation I had never dealt with before. I could give the instructions for an unconscious or suspended patient without even glancing at the screen, but definitely not for a choking patient. AMPDS isn't always perfect for categorizing calls, but as far as giving instructions goes, I can't fault it. After telling it the child's age, current condition and what the nursery staff had already done, it told me that the next thing they should try was to straddle the child (who was now collapsed on the floor) and give an abdominal thrust from above. I passed this on to the nursery nurse, who instructed the child's mother to do that. It's not often that you get to tell people to punch a toddler in the stomach! She did this, making a delightful squidging sound, and the nursery nurse went to inspect the outcome.

'He looks a little less blue ... yes, I can see that he's breathing!' she exclaimed.

I told her to look in the little boy's mouth and fish out the offending rice cake. This she did.

'Youch!' she cried. 'He bit me! Oh well, I suppose that's a good sign ...'

At this point the toddler started to cry.

'Oh, thank God for that!' said the nursery nurse. 'I've never been so happy to hear a child crying!'

Suddenly she burst into tears and so did the child's mother. It's not often you hear people crying with relief/happiness so I even started to feel a bit misty eyed myself. I was really glad that they waited until the child was okay to fall to pieces. Actually, this is something I have noticed before – people crack up and are useless when their parent is the patient, but when it's their child they somehow manage to hold it together and do as they are told. Perhaps it's some kind of primitive instinct that makes us protect our offspring, whereas we expect to be protected by our parents. Anyway, it was a couple more minutes until the ambulance arrived, so I had a nice chat with the nursery nurse as she pulled herself together. She asked for my name – perhaps the nursery will send me a thank-you letter. I hope so. I have never had a thank-you letter before – and if someone sends you one, you get your name in LAS news!

# Help Me!

8 June 2006

Me: AMBULANCE SERVICE, WHAT'S THE PROBLEM? TELL ME EXACTLY
WHAT HAPPENED.
Her: IT'S MY ELDERLY FATHER. HE'S HAVING TROUBLE WITH HIS
BREATHING AND I CAN'T WAKE HIM UP.

Me: OKAY. WHAT'S THE ADDRESS OF THE EMERGENCY?
Her: 10 FOREST VILLAS, RICHMOND.

Me: NOW I NEED TO ASK YOU A FEW QUESTIONS, BUT THIS WON'T
DELAY HELP COMING.
Her: BUT I DON'T HAVE TIME TO ANSWER QUESTIONS! PLEASE,
HELP ME!

Me: I NEED TO ASK YOU QUESTIONS SO I KNOW EXACTLY WHAT IS
GOING ON, THEN I CAN TELL YOU WHAT TO DO. WHILE I AM DOING
THAT, SOMEONE ELSE IS ARRANGING THE AMBULANCE.
Her: I CAN'T *DO* ANYTHING! JUST GET HELP HERE.

Me: HELP *IS* BEING ARRANGED. HOW OLD IS HE?
Her: HOW *OLD?* WHAT DOES THAT MATTER? HE'S UNCONSCIOUS!

Me: APPROXIMATELY EIGHTY? OLDER? YOUNGER?
Her: HE'S EIGHTY-TWO! PLEASE, HELP!

Me: NOW, YOU'VE SAID HE'S NOT CONSCIOUS. BUT IS HE BREATHING?
Her: YES, NO, I DON'T KNOW! JUST HELP!

(I select the cardiac arrest card, because our protocols state that if
someone is unconscious and the caller is on the scene but can't confirm that they *are* breathing, we treat them as if they are not.)

Me: NOW, STAY ON THE LINE. I AM GOING TO TELL YOU WHAT TO DO
   NEXT. LIE HIM FLAT ON THE GROUND.
Her: I CAN'T DO THAT!

Me: OKAY, IS THERE SOMEONE YOU CAN GET TO HELP YOU?
Her: MY HUSBAND IS HERE.

Me: OKAY, ASK YOUR HUSBAND TO HELP YOU. LIE YOUR FATHER FLAT
   ON HIS BACK, WITHOUT ANY PILLOWS, THEN KNEEL NEXT TO HIM
   AND CHECK IN HIS MOUTH FOR ANY FOOD OR VOMIT.
Her: THAT WON'T WORK!

Me: THAT'S WHAT YOU NEED TO DO. ASK YOUR HUSBAND FOR HELP. DO
   IT NOW, I'LL STAY ON THE PHONE.
Her: I CAN'T! HELP ME!

Me: I AM HELPING YOU. THIS IS WHAT YOU NEED TO DO. GO AND DO IT
   NOW AND COME BACK TO THE PHONE WHEN IT'S DONE.
Her: BUT HE'S IN A WHEELCHAIR. WHERE IS THE AMBULANCE? MAKE
   THEM HURRY UP!

Me: THE AMBULANCE IS DRIVING TO YOU ON BLUE LIGHTS, I CAN'T
   MAKE THEM COME ANY FASTER. WHAT I CAN DO IS TELL YOU HOW
   TO HELP HIM UNTIL THE AMBULANCE CREW GET THERE. PLEASE, ASK
   YOUR HUSBAND TO HELP YOU GET YOUR FATHER OUT OF THE CHAIR
   AND ON TO THE FLOOR.

(In the background I hear her, very reluctantly, talking to her husband: 'She says we need to get him out of the chair ... no, I don't
think ... I've told her that it's urgent but she's not listening ...
expects us to deal with it ourselves.' I don't have time to set her
straight – with every second her father is getting closer to death.)

Her: I CAN'T DO IT!
Me: RIGHT, WE'RE GOING TO HAVE TO WORK ON HIM IN THE CHAIR,
   THEN. PUT ONE HAND BEHIND HIS NECK, THE OTHER ON HIS
   FOREHEAD, TILT HIS HEAD BACK AND SEE IF YOU CAN HEAR OR
   FEEL ANY BREATHING. DO THAT NOW AND TELL ME WHAT YOU FIND.

Her: NOTHING. HE'S NOT BREATHING. PLEASE, PLEASE HELP ME!

Me: WE NEED TO START RESUSCITATION. ARE YOU *SURE* YOU CAN'T GET
  HIM OUT OF THE CHAIR?

Her: I'VE TOLD YOU, I CAN'T DO THAT!
Me: OKAY, WE'LL DO IT IN THE CHAIR.

(This is probably going to do as much good as not doing CPR
at all, but to stop at this stage would be to concede defeat. Even
if circumstances dictate that effective CPR cannot be performed,
it is better to do something and let the relative feel they have done
all they can to help, rather than just stand there and wait for the
ambulance.)

Me: PUT THE HEEL OF YOUR HAND ON THE BREASTBONE, RIGHT
  BETWEEN THE NIPPLES. PRESS DOWN ...

At this point the ambulance crew arrives. I've been on the phone
for six minutes – double the average time the brain can survive
undamaged without breathing or CPR – and we've done nothing
in the way of resus at all.

# More Bananas

Banana Man is getting totally out of control. I think he actually spent about six hours solidly dialling 999 last night, informing us that some combination of the following was occurring.

- He's at 10 Bethnal Green Road.

- He's on the runway at Gatwick Airport.

- He's at Buckingham Palace (this is a new one).

- He's at London City Airport (he must have figured Gatwick is out of our area).

- He's itchy.

- He's feeling dizzy.

- His girlfriend is itchy/feeling dizzy.

- He'd like a banana.

- He'd like us to have a banana.

- He wants a carrot (another new one).

I have tried *everything* to stop him calling. I have tried telling him that he is wasting our time and preventing real calls from getting through. I have tried telling him he is breaking the law and that we will trace him and prosecute him. I have tried pretending he is genuine and taking the call normally in the hope he will lose his nerve and cancel the ambulance. Nothing works. I've given up and noted his number on a piece of paper, and as soon as I see it appear on my screen, I cut the line straight away. Something seriously has to be done. I am at the end of my tether.

Banana Man went to sleep at 2 a.m. tonight. You could tell because the call rate suddenly dropped considerably.

# Plenty Womiting

'What's the problem?' I asked.

'I called you earlier!' said an angry-sounding man. 'It's Mr Bloggs! From 14 Gravida House, Bile Street, E20!' He sounded very angry that I didn't know who he was. I looked up the original call. It was from a twenty-year-old lady – the caller's girlfriend – six weeks pregnant, vomiting. It had been through CTA, who had decreed this was a bit of garden-variety morning sickness and that we were not to send an ambulance. CTA had given home care advice, and told the caller that if she really wanted to go to hospital, she should make her own way. I repeated this back to the caller, to make sure he'd understood the CTA paramedic properly and see why he was calling back.

'Yes!' he said. 'We are at the hospital!'

'Erm,' I said, confused. 'So why are you calling 999?'

'Because they say we have to wait to be seen! And she is womiting! You must tell them to see us straight away!'

'I'm afraid I can't do that,' I said (not adding that even if I could, I wouldn't be doing anything of the sort). 'There are always long waits in hospital, you will just have to wait with everyone else. If you have any problems, speak to the hospital staff!'

The man continued ranting and saying that CTA had assured him that he would be seen immediately (which I am sure is a lie!) and that it was disgusting and didn't I know that his girlfriend was WOMITING? We are not usually allowed to hang up on callers, but if they are ringing from an A&E department we can make an exception, so I took great pleasure in telling him: 'Sir, I have four calls waiting to be answered, and these people could be dying, so I am going to have to terminate this call. Goodbye!'

# Goodbye

## 1 July 2006

On Thursday night I took a call from an extremely upset lady who had been woken in the night by her elderly husband having a fit. He had never had one before, which I took as a rather bad sign – if a fitting patient isn't epileptic, alcoholic, diabetic or a child with a fever, then it generally means something is badly wrong with them.

I stayed on the line with her and tried to calm her down as we waited for the fit to stop.

'Why is it taking so long?' she wailed. I looked at the clock – we'd been on the phone for two minutes and thirty seconds. I strongly suspected that, unless there happened to be an ambulance parked outside her house last time she'd called, it just hadn't seemed that long. The longest minutes on earth are those spent waiting with a critically ill loved-one.

The fit stopped, and the lady laid her husband on his side. I crossed my fingers that he would start breathing. I heard a snoring sound, which at first sounded encouraging (people usually snore post-fit) but the snoring became increasingly irregular and the sounds stranger. I strongly suspected that I was listening to agonal breathing.

I think the lady knew what was happening. She totally lost it at that stage and put the phone to one side, so I couldn't talk to her. I could hear her in the background, sobbing and saying, 'Oh Jim, oh sweetheart, please don't go. Come on, darling, please stay, please stay ...' and I could hear her kissing his forehead.

Meanwhile, I was shouting 'PICK UP THE PHONE, PLEEEASE!' at the top of my voice, trying to get her attention.

After a few seconds this worked, and I began the instructions to put the patient on his back to check for breathing.

'I don't think … yes … no … he's gone blue … oh no, he's … yes, he is breathing … no, I don't know …'

I tried to use the 'breath timer' gadget, but it was no use, she was sobbing too much. I asked her to put the phone to her husband's mouth, so I could listen to his breathing myself. She did so. There was nothing. I couldn't hear anything.

At this point the crew arrived. I heard one of them say to the patient 'Can you open your eyes?' (which I thought was promising, because it's what ambulance crews say to unconscious people) and not 'When did you last see him?' (which is what they say to the relatives of dead people). Then one of the crew came to the phone.

'Hi, we're here …' she said, '… and I think we're going to need a second crew.'

I didn't need to ask the reason why a second crew was required. We always send two to suspended patients if we can.

Half an hour later the patient was blued into hospital, still suspended.

I suppose it is better that she got to say goodbye to her husband with a kiss on the head than by having to thump his chest and breathe into his mouth.

# Observation Shift II

5 July 2006

Last time I went out with Steve and his crewmate I found that whatever I wished for, we got sent to. Since I had wished for some nasty trauma and a cardiac arrest, it was a busy day. This time I wished for a nice little old lady who'd fallen over and, again, this was precisely what we got. In Control terms, this is about as simple as you can get. It is non-life-threatening (so you do not have to bust a gut getting someone there) but it is also a valid call – as soon as someone is available, off they go. But I was about to discover that something simple for us is not so simple for an ambulance crew.

Elaine, aged eighty, has lived alone in her house since the death of her husband. Her younger friend, Sandra, comes to visit every day and helps out with the shopping. She also has meals on wheels and a home help. Despite having arthritis, bilateral knee replacements, heart trouble, mild confusion and depression, she gets by. On this bitterly cold morning she was getting out her electric fire and, carrying it to her bedside, slipped over. She fell awkwardly against the bed and an agonizing pain shot through her right leg.

Luckily Elaine had fallen by the phone, so she was quick to summon help. Not wanting to bother the emergency services so early in the morning, she rang Sandra. Sandra had come straight round, but after a quick examination she had realized that Elaine had hurt herself badly in the fall and that an ambulance was needed. Enter us.

Elaine was in good spirits and not a lot of pain when we arrived. Her sense of humour was intact – she was laughing at herself for falling – and she was very apologetic about calling us out. (The genuine callers always are.) I wondered if it was going to be an 'assist only' job, where the crew lift the patient, put her back to bed and make her a cup of tea. However, as Steve straightened Elaine's legs, I could see clearly that one was shorter than the other and drooping to one side – a clear indicator of a broken hip.

Seeing the concern on our faces, Elaine became worried. 'What is it? What have I done?'

'I'm afraid,' said Steve, 'you've broken your hip.'

'Oh!' said Elaine, relief coursing across her face. 'Is that all?'

I wondered what she thought we were going to say.

Now came the difficult and unpleasant part. With the aid of some Entonox (pain-relieving gas), we tried to assist Elaine into the carry chair so we could get her downstairs and into the ambulance. But the slightest movement had her in complete agony. The gas seemed to be making her confused too, and she forgot what had happened to her and kept yelling out: 'What's happened to me? What could be causing all this pain? I have never felt this uncomfortable in MY ENTIRE LIFE!' She was shaking and turning terribly white. It wasn't pleasant to watch. As Control staff you are generally distanced from people's pain. You get all the emotional upset and the lurid descriptions of gory events, but the physical pain is something you don't think about. You tend to think: 'Broken hip … non-life-threatening, simple' – without really getting your head around what it is like to have one. Elaine's agony is something I will remember every time I take a 'broken hip' call.

Once we stopped trying to move Elaine, her pain subsided somewhat and she returned to being the cheery old lady we'd first encountered and apologized profusely for 'being a big baby'. Meanwhile, Steve's crewmate, who is a paramedic, decided Entonox alone was not enough to get Elaine out of here. It was time to bring in the big guns. He fired up a vial of morphine and injected it into Elaine. Then we sat around a bit and waited for it to work. Sandra conducted some breathing exercises while I helped pack up Elaine's belongings. Eventually Elaine started going a bit woozy and getting a big grin on her face, and we were able to lift her into the carry chair. There was a lot of hollering as we moved her, but this was immediately followed by relief from everyone as we all announced: 'Well, that's the worst bit done! Off to the hospital!'

It had taken over an hour to get her into the ambulance.

By now, Elaine was away with the fairies. Steve tried to get her to give a score to her pain. Earlier, she'd given it nine out of ten.

'Oh,' she said, flapping her arms dismissively. 'Hardly anything!'

'I need a number,' said Steve.

'Erm, I really don't know,' said Elaine. 'I can't remember any numbers!'

'Elaine,' smiled Steve, 'I'm not taking you anywhere until you give me a number!'

'Um ... sixteen!' announced Elaine, and broke into fits of giggles.

Steve gave up at this point and we went off to the hospital.

I am sure Elaine will be fine, although it is clear her bones aren't what they used to be, and perhaps she will have to give up living in a two-storey house by herself. It is sad that such a lovely person – who is so cheerful and friendly and has clearly lived such a full and rich life – has ended up being let down by her own body, and even sadder to think that, whatever I achieve with my life, more or less the same will happen to me. I shall never look at 'old woman on the floor' as just a simple, boring call again.

The next few calls were less interesting – a man who was drunk in a pub (how unusual), an assault victim who'd run away by the time we'd arrived, and a maternataxi.

We then had a bit of a mystery call. All we got down the MDT was '30-year-old male, ? cardiac arrest'. I felt excited and horrified at the same time – if the patient was thirty years old, there would almost certainly be a resuscitation attempt, which I desperately wanted to see. But at the same time, the death of a young person would be a horrible thing to witness, something that might haunt me for years.

Then the phone rang. It was Control.

'Bit of a strange one here! We're not sure what's going on. A woman has just called saying that someone told her that her son is dead in his flat ... but she's not sure of his address. We think it's 116 Long Road in SW5 ... there's definitely a six in the number ... could you stand by for confirmation? ... Yes, it's definitely 116. Flat 8. The police are on their way.'

I had a lot of thoughts at once. The first was that I knew the type of call we were going to – the kind when someone mutters unintelligible nonsense about someone being dead and you have to send an ambulance just to find that they aren't dead. The second was that if someone was suspended, they'd certainly be dead by the time we'd tried every house in Long Road that has a six in it. The third was, how the hell can you not know your son's address?

Then we were outside 116 Long Road. Knocking at the door yielded no answer, perhaps unsurprisingly. Corpses don't generally open doors. The police pulled up seconds later and one of the officers aimed his steel-toecapped boot at the door. It swung open with minimal effort. (Burglars, I recommend you give that house a go.) Two police officers and three ambulance people trooped up the stairs and knocked on the door of Flat 8. There was no reply, so the policeman took aim once again. Just as he was poised for the kick, the door creaked open, almost causing the policeman to fall horizontally through, as if in a comedy sketch.

A bleary-eyed, dark-skinned man stood there in his boxer shorts, looking bemused.

'Are you Peter Jones?' enquired the policeman.

'No ...' said the man.

'Your parents rang us, they were worried about you.'

'My parents are in Brazil!'

The police officers exchanged glances. 'I think we have the wrong house,' said one.

'I think we do,' agreed the other. 'Well, he's definitely not dead. Sorry to bother you, sir. Goodnight.'

And we all trooped out again. We did try all the other houses in Long Road with a six in them, but none of them had a Flat 8. So it was that we conceded defeat and returned to our vehicles. I felt kind of guilty that I was actually disappointed to have found the occupant alive and well.

# Back to Control

The first thing I did on my return was to check the call-taking logs to see if the parents of the 'possibly dead' young man in Long Road rang back. They never did. So it's possible that, somewhere in Chelsea, a body is still festering! Of course it's far more likely that the call was a hoax, or that the mother was completely over-reacting and the son was alive and well.

Management said they are pleased that I have been volunteering for observation shifts and that it will stand me in good stead for promotion. I have asked them if I can do more shifts upstairs on the dispatch desks, and hopefully — at some point in the distant future — become an allocator. Having concluded that my driving may never reach the required standard for a paramedic, I think this is the best way forward for me.

I feel like I'm an old hand at call taking and I'm ready for a new challenge soon.

# Brenda Banned

Brenda Kramer has been prosecuted! There is an injunction preventing her from ever calling 999 again! It is all over the local papers. Apparently she made over 1,000 calls over the last 3 years, at a cost to the taxpayer of *nearly £250,000!* That would have paid for HEMS to go out 250 times or have covered 10 EMDs' salaries for a whole year! An Ambulance Service spokesman said that regular callers misusing the service cost an estimated £5 million a year. Just think what that would pay for! Anyway, Brenda was given a 28-day suspended sentence, and if she ever rings again, she could go to prison. If she has a genuine emergency, she has to call her daughter, who will call on her behalf. I don't know what will happen if she can't get hold of her daughter. It would be ironic if she couldn't get an ambulance when she genuinely needed one because of all the times she'd cried wolf. I have to say, it would serve her right. Countless people must have suffered because of her misuse of the service – I have no sympathy for the woman.

# Bystanders from Hell

## 21 July 2006

There was a massive road traffic accident on the A21 in Bromley today. There were five cars involved, one of which ended up on its side and another in a ditch. It was a miracle that no one was seriously hurt. Because it was near a school and a row of shops, we must have taken at least twenty-five calls on it. It's funny the way the reactions of the bystanders and their levels of helpfulness vary. Some will give you every detail you need and practically rescue the patients themselves while others seem to think you ought to be grateful that they've called at all, even if they don't give you any useful information.

We all agreed that the ultimate nightmare-bystander-caller's routine goes something like this.

1. Ring 999, even though you can see at least four people doing the same. If you happen to be passing on a bus or car, and have no idea where you are, do this anyway, and under no circumstances get off the bus to help, as this may make you late for an important engagement, such as a church service.
2. Swear repeatedly at the call taker for asking you stupid questions such as 'What's happened?' and 'Where are you?' Hang up the phone. If the call taker is impertinent enough to ring you back again, switch the phone off.
3. Refuse to follow first-aid instructions such as controlling bleeding and doing CPR – those are the Ambulance Service's job! Put the patient in the recovery position, even though he is fully conscious and has a broken arm.
4. Switch the phone back on and ring the Ambulance Service to berate them for not being there yet. You rang two whole

minutes ago! Become stunned at the incompetence of the call taker when you tell him you're ringing about 'the accident outside Tesco' and he does not instantly realize which call you mean out of the 200 calls taken in the last hour. Hang up again.

5. Give the patient a cup of tea and a cigarette. Stand back as the patient starts to vomit.

6. Flag down a police patrol car. Tell the police you called for an ambulance half an hour ago but none has arrived. The police ring Ambulance Control, who have no record of the call but have been trying to contact a person who rang about 'an accident outside Tesco' five minutes ago, but whose mobile phone seems to be malfunctioning and repeatedly dropping the call.

7. The ambulance arrives. Yell at the ambulance crew for taking too long. Tell them how to do their job, as you read in *Metro* lately that all ambulances are staffed by technicians who have no training.

8. Go home and tell everyone how dreadful the Ambulance Service were and how the patient would never have survived without your intervention. Sell the story to the local newspaper. Be acclaimed as a local hero.

# A Sad Suspended

## 28 July 2006

I knew it was going to be a suspended the second the operator connected the call. While a hysterical caller does not always (or even usually) mean a serious call, these weren't the usual panicking screams but howls of sheer terror. I wondered if it was going to be something gruesome. It was almost a relief when she told me that the patient was her elderly grandmother, who was 'not waking up'.

'Hurry up!' she sobbed, again and again, oblivious of the fact that she hadn't even given me an address to send the ambulance to. It's usually one of the most frustrating things on earth to be told to hurry when you are waiting for a response from the caller, but I could hardly feel annoyed in the circumstances. I managed to coax the address out of her (thankfully, just down the road from Tottenham Ambulance Station) and confirm what I'd already guessed – that the patient was not breathing. This flagged the call as a red, and already two ambulances and an FRU were on their way. Now for the hard bit – giving CPR instruction to someone who was barely together enough to remember where she was.

'Did you see what happened?' is the next question. This helps us determine whether it's going to be a 'working job' or a 'purple plus' and therefore how much we should try to coax a reluctant caller into giving CPR. This caller, unfortunately, did not see what happened – she'd just come to visit, she sobbed, and found her grandmother in the bed. Not a good sign – she could have been there for hours. But there was still a remote chance, so I ploughed on with the 'get the patient on her back, check the airway, check for breathing ...' instructions. It took a little while because the caller was sobbing so much, but she was doing as she was told – she wanted to do everything she could to save her grandmother. Once she had confirmed that the patient was not breathing, I moved on to the CPR instructions.

'I'm going to tell you how to do resuscitation,' I began. 'Put the heel of your hand . . .'

'No!' sobbed the caller, who had been totally compliant until now. 'I can't, I can't, just send the ambulance!'

This was a setback.

'Yes, you can – I can tell you how. We need to do this to give her the best chance,' I said, which is my usual coaxing patter.

'No,' she said, 'I can't.'

This time I understood that she didn't mean, 'I can't, I'm too scared, I don't know how,' but, 'I can't, it's too late, she's already dead.' I didn't mention the CPR again, but stayed on the line with her anyway, even though I had nothing left to say or do other than ooze meaningless platitudes such as, 'Help will be with you soon,' and, 'You did very well, you did everything you could.' Now the urgency was over, I became aware of a background noise that I'd been blotting out. There was a small child crying in the background.

'Is that a child with you?' I asked.

'Yes . . . my little brother,' she told me. The boy was wailing inconsolably and shouting 'Granny!' and the caller's name. He sounded about five. It occurred to me at that point that, to have a brother that young, my caller was most likely not an adult yet herself.

'Okay, let's get him out of there,' I said. 'Both of you leave the front door open and go and stand outside and wait for the ambulance. Give your little brother a hug and look after him.' They both sounded terrified, I figured they needed each other.

I didn't say anything else, but I heard the girl explaining that because she couldn't wake Grandma up, she thought she was gone (not 'dead', never 'dead'). The little boy howled that he didn't want Grandma to go, and the girl said that she didn't either, and then they both cried again. Then a familiar sound – *nee naw nee naw nee naw* – it was the FRU arriving. The girl snatched up the phone and thanked me about ten times before going to greet it. I wasn't sure what she was thanking me for – in retrospect I think it was the fact that I'd got an ambulance there so that she didn't have to be the responsible adult any more.

# Heart Problem

1 August 2006

Me: AMBULANCE SERVICE, TELL ME EXACTLY WHAT'S HAPPENED ...

Old lady: HELLO, DEAR. I'M SORRY TO BOTHER YOU, BUT I THINK THERE'S A PROBLEM WITH MY HEART.

Me: (TYPES.) I SEE. AND WHAT'S THE ADDRESS?

Old lady: IT'S 29 FLOWERPOT COTTAGES IN SUTTON.

Me: AND HOW OLD ARE YOU?

Old lady: I'M NINETY-THREE.

Me: OKAY. WHAT SYMPTOMS ARE YOU HAVING?

Old lady: WELL, YOU SEE ... I'M NOT EXACTLY HAVING ANY SYMPTOMS. IT'S JUST ... I'M WORRIED THAT MY HEART MIGHT HAVE STOPPED BEATING.

Me: STOPPED BEATING?

Old lady: YES ... I CAN'T FEEL THE PULSE AT ALL! I'VE TRIED BOTH WRISTS AND MY NECK AND MY CHEST AND THERE'S NOTHING THERE AT ALL!

Me: ERRRR ... BUT YOUR HEART *MUST* BE BEATING ... BECAUSE YOU'RE TALKING TO ME. IF YOUR HEART STOPS BEATING, YOU DIE.

Old lady: I KNOW THAT, DEAR. THAT'S WHY I RANG!

Me: I MEAN, YOU DIE STRAIGHT AWAY.

Old lady: OH! SO YOU MEAN, IT IS STILL BEATING?

Me: YES. IF YOU DON'T BELIEVE ME, I CAN SEND ONE OF MY NICE AMBULANCE CREWS ROUND, AND THEY CAN ATTACH YOU TO A HEART MONITOR AND SHOW YOU ON A BIG SCREEN.

Old lady: REALLY? OH NO, IT WON'T BE NECESSARY. I DON'T WANT TO WASTE THEIR TIME. THANK YOU, DEAR, I FEEL MUCH BETTER NOW.

# Where Are the Regulars?

I must admit that I have quite missed Brenda Kramer. I did not think I ever wanted to hear her voice again but, now that she's stopped calling, night shifts just aren't the same. I wonder what she is doing with her time?

I have not taken a call from Sally Wiltshire for ages either. I remember what she said about the doctors not expecting her to live past her twenty-fifth birthday, which was about ten months ago now. It was a quiet night shift tonight, so I did a search on the computer system to see if we'd taken any calls to her address lately. Nothing. The last call was back in February. I hope she isn't dead. I hope she's finally got help, made the friends she so desperately wanted and doesn't feel the need to call us any more.

At least we still have Banana Man. He's still calling us relentlessly every night. We're under instructions to hang up as soon as we have identified a caller as being him. I do so with pleasure.

# Common Beliefs Held by the General Public About Calling 999

Life would be so much easier if everyone in the world knew how the Ambulance Service and the 999 call-taking system worked. I've had a particularly frustrating day where all the callers seem to be labouring under a variety of misapprehensions which I have listed below. If only there was time during a 999 call to set them straight ...

1. The LOUDER you shout, the faster the ambulance will come.
2. The faster you speak, the faster the ambulance will come.
3. Even though the call taker asked for the address of the emergency, what he really wants to hear is a detailed description of what happened, starting with the patient having his tonsils out in 1962.
4. The ambulance cannot possibly leave the ambulance station until you hang up, so it is imperative to hang up as soon as possible, even if the call taker is trying to tell you something. Hanging up several times will make the ambulance come twice as fast.
5. A good call taker should just take the address and send the ambulance. A bad call taker will find out what has happened, prioritize the call and give you instructions on what to do next, thus wasting precious time when you could have been running around the house screaming.
6. The call taker will never have taken a 999 call before so they need to be told that a man under a truck is a 'serious emergency' and that the ambulance 'had better get here quick'. (Or, more commonly, that a 29-year-old with belly ache is a

'serious emergency' and that the ambulance 'had better get here quick').

7. There is only one person who works for the Ambulance Service. That person takes the call and then jumps in the ambulance. If you call back, the person you speak to will know exactly which of the 3,500-plus daily calls you are talking about without you giving them irrelevant details such as the address.

8. The Ambulance Service have an ambulance parked at the end of every road, enabling them to reach any location within thirty seconds. If they take longer than this to reach an emergency, it is due to incompetence and slacking.

9. If you don't know the answer to a question, provide an irrelevant piece of information instead: Q: 'Is he changing colour?' A: 'He's in a lot of pain.' Q: 'Has she passed out?' A: 'She is upstairs.' Q: 'Is she conscious?' A: 'She's a black woman.'

10. 'Conscious' and 'unconscious' mean exactly the same thing. Common causes of unconsciousness include: being in too much pain to talk, Alzheimer's disease, being a bit upset.

11. Call takers work for British Telecom, they know nothing about medical stuff or ambulances, but a lot about switchboards. They also have the phone number for your local hospital, GP, Social Services, Pizza Hut …

12. Never say 'please' or 'thank you' – call takers find this highly insulting and will cancel the ambulance and send you the police instead.

# Going Upstairs

Management have decided that from now on, I am to work primarily on the dispatch desks, upstairs. This is good news careerwise – upstairs is where the more experienced, knowledgeable people work and where the important decisions are made, so it means that Management must be impressed with my work. I'd really love to become an allocator at some point – knowing I have the responsibility to decide which calls get the ambulance would be fantastic! Even better, I now have a seat by a window and twenty-minute breaks instead of fifteen-minute ones!

First of all I am going to be trained as a radio operator and then I will learn how to allocate. If all goes well, I can apply for an allocator position in a year's time. For the moment, though, I have the lowly dispatcher's spot. I am doing a lot of arranging of GPs and a lot of ringing people back to advise of delays. In other words, I am talking to a lot of timewasters right now.

I have been allocated to the south-east desk (although I will be doing shifts now and then on all the sectors, so I get to know them all). The main allocator there is Jenny, who has been here for fifteen years and has seen and heard everything. She does not stand for any nonsense from anyone – patients, crews or Management – and I think this is a good way to be. The Radio Op here is Snowy. She is nineteen years old and likes shoes and holidays, both of which are excellent topics to fill long and boring night shifts, so we get on well. At the moment it is just the three of us on the desk permanently – there is a vacancy for an allocator, which gets filled by random people who are in on overtime. They will be advertising the post in a few months. Maybe, if all goes well, I could be the one to get it.

# How the Dispatch Area Works

2 September 2006

Upstairs from the call-taking pit is the dispatch area. It is generally regarded as a privilege to work in the dispatch area for the following reasons.

1. They have windows.
2. They have better heating.
3. No one is rude to you (except Management).

The dispatch area is split into six sector desks, each covering a different geographical part of London and the ambulance stations therein. (Note: Ambulances, contrary to popular belief, are not based at hospitals, although many ambulance stations are near hospitals.)

When fully manned, each desk has four people working on it: two allocators, a radio operator and a dispatcher. The allocator is in charge of the desk and makes all the important decisions such as which ambulance goes to which call and whether ambulances should be sent to calls (if, for instance, the crew get covered in vomit and their carry chair won't open). I've picked up some tips about allocating already from peering over the shoulder of Jenny, our desk's allocator. She has a screen that shows all the outstanding calls. As soon as a call taker has an address, details of the call appear on Jenny's screen, and it is updated with more details every time the call taker presses 'return'. As soon as she has enough information, she can send the call details to an ambulance. She also has to make sure other people both within the Ambulance Service and elsewhere are told about the call. She might need to tell HEMS – if it's a call about a serious injury – or an ambulance manager

(DSO), Management within the control room, the police, the fire brigade, the coastguard, London Transport, the RSPCA, the Gas Board ...

To send call details to an ambulance, she just presses a button on her computer keyboard and the call appears on a screen (the MDT) in the ambulance. The MDT rings like a phone to alert the crew and, as the call taker continues taking information, the crew gets regular updates. The crew will know everything you've told the call taker – and they will also know if you are rude to them or won't answer their questions, because the call taker will be sure to make a note of it on the ticket for all to see!

Everyone in Control also has a computer screen in front of them that shows a map of London embellished with a triangle for each call and a cartoon ambulance for every ambulance. The ambulances move in real time and, by hovering over them with your mouse, you can see which direction they are travelling in and how fast they are going (although they always appear to be pointing to the right, so sometimes they look like they are going backwards). Or, if they are stationary, you can see when they last moved. As well as using this information to get ambulances to calls faster and to assist them in finding their patients, you can also use it to spy on crews and watch them pop to McDonald's to get their lunch. If something goes wrong with the MDT, you can get 'ghost' ambulances on the mapping system. For months there was an ambulance 'stuck' in a reservoir near Tottenham. When, six months ago, an FRU was involved in a high-speed collision and caught fire (miraculously, no one was seriously hurt), its cartoon remained frozen at the spot of the accident for ever – the ghost of a dead ambulance. When other ambulances break down, you can see where they've gone to be repaired – the 'ambulance hospital' just outside London. And sometimes when London Ambulance sell their vehicles to other ambulance services, you can see them bobbing around the map in their new homes. There's quite a few in Essex – and I've even spotted one in Lancashire!

The radio operator talks to ambulance crews on the radio, for instance to help them if they get lost or ring back patients if they want more information about the call. Being the radio operator is quite fun, although I'm quite new to it. I like it because most of the ambulance crews are friendly (though they do have a tendency to all talk at once and ask silly questions such as, 'Are we the near-est to this call you've sent us on?' to which I am tempted to reply, 'No, there's another crew at the end of the road but you looked like you needed the exercise!'). A lot of the time the radio operator acts as go-between, facilitating communication between ambu-lance crew and patient. If there's any more information the crew want, the radio operator rings the patient. Most queries are due to ambulances not being able to find locations. It is amazing how many people, despite being told to meet the ambulance, stay inside and just expect the crew to automatically find them. A lot of addresses in London are in rabbit warren-like estates and not all houses are clearly numbered. Delays are caused every day because crews simply can't find the place they are going to. It also surprises me how often someone will call 999 on their mobile and then switch it off or not answer when we call them back.

The dispatcher is the most junior person on the desk and does all the long-winded tasks such as finding out which crews are using which ambulances at the beginning of the shifts, ringing up GPs to arrange home visits and ringing round the hospitals to try and find out where patients have escaped from. They also have to ring back patients if there is going to be a delay sending an ambulance, which is my least favourite task _ever_. I hate being the bearer of bad news. If the patient is seriously ill, I feel guilty for letting them down, even though it's not really my fault that other people are ill too and the ambulances are all with them. If I think the call is a load of rubbish – which a lot of them are – I have difficulty biting my tongue and not telling the caller that. We are not allowed to tell someone that they are misusing the service or that they should be making their own way to hospital.

It feels very different working upstairs after two years of call taking. Last week I felt like I knew everything about the art of ambulance control, now I feel like I'm the newbie again. It's nice to be part of a small, close-knit team on the desk – call taking can be a bit lonely sometimes. Chatting with the crews and my deskmates makes the job a lot less stressful. I was worried at first that working upstairs would be boring, because I'm not as close to the action, but in fact it's even more exciting. I get to follow every call from the second the phone rings to the point where the crew arrive at hospital, and I also get to find out what happens to some of the patients. I can listen to the 999 calls and talk to the crews who treated the patient. Best of all, I am involved in the decision-making process. Every call is different up here, and it's not just a matter of following protocols any more – we really have to use our brains.

# Banana Man Foiled

I am pleased to report that finally, after six months of torment, Banana Man has been caught and stopped. I worked for twelve hours on the east central desk today and there was *not one* single call to that particular Woolworth's, no one collapsed on the runway at Gatwick Airport, no itchy penises and definitely no offers of a banana. He was caught by an ingenious police officer, who called him back and pretended to be someone running a competition, asking him to give his name and address so his prize could be sent. Banana Man took the bait and revealed all.

It transpired that Banana Man is only a teenager and is seriously disabled, so at the moment he isn't being prosecuted. Social Services are getting involved and trying to put a stop to the calls – and so far, so good. I must admit that after months of tearing my hair out and feeling terrorized and frustrated by this individual, my sympathy-o-meter is rating about a zero and I am not terribly impressed by this lenient attitude. Disabled or not, he had the presence of mind to go out and acquire a new SIM card each time one was cut off, and he was with-it enough to answer call takers' questions and laugh when they reprimanded him for hoaxing. I just don't believe that he was totally unaware of the consequences of his actions, and I think he should receive some kind of punishment for it. It also begs the question – if he is young and/or disabled, where were his parents or carers when the calls were being made?

Still, I suppose this is not for me to worry about and I should just be grateful that I will never be driven to distraction by him again. I expect to see a sharp decrease in the number of calls recorded in the east central area from now on.

# The Most Annoying Diagnosis
# in the World

17 September 2006

Do you know what the most annoying diagnosis in the world is? I'll tell you. It's people who ring in because *they can't sleep!* Specifically, people who ring in at 4 a.m., moaning about their insomnia, when you are in the middle of your first painful night shift and are propping your eyes open with matchsticks. When you would most dearly like to sleep but aren't allowed to. I feel like saying: 'Well, you can't sleep and I can't stay awake! How about you come and do my job while I go to bed? I promise that after doing this all night, you will be so exhausted that you will sleep like a log!'

# Dognap

18 September 2006

Today I nearly broke into a patient's house and stole his dog.

Okay, that sounds bad. Maybe I'd better start from the beginning. The call came from the police, and read:

**NEIGHBOURS CONCERNED FOR ELDERLY GENTLEMAN. HE HAS NOT BEEN SEEN FOR A FEW DAYS AND HIS DOG IS WHINING AT THE WINDOW.**

Calls like this are called 'suspected collapse behind locked doors'. Half the time we go to them and find a dead body on the other side of the locked door, the rest of the time we find a very angry person returning from a shopping trip to find their front door hanging off its hinges as the police search their house fruitlessly. This call, however, was neither. The elderly man had fallen and had been on the floor for an unspecified length of time. His house was in a revolting state, the crew had to step over a dead rat to get to him. The dog – a small, skinny creature of unspecified breed – did not look as if it had been receiving the best of care. The owner admitted that he just couldn't look after it any more – in fact, he couldn't even look after himself. He begged the crew to find someone to look after it.

The crew were now posed with a problem: they needed to get the patient into hospital straight away, but didn't want to leave the dog. In the end, they felt they had no option but to leave it to us to arrange something for the dog while they rushed the patient in. The police secured the house, leaving the dog alone inside. And then we spent the rest of the day trying to arrange help for the dog. Getting a dog rescued is not as easy as it sounds. The RSPCA can't take it away just like that, the police can't help, it was impossible to contact any relatives ... we didn't know what else to try.

It was getting towards the end of the day and the thought of that little dog whining at the window was beginning to haunt me in a way that even the most horrific human calls fail to. I couldn't sleep knowing it was slowing starving and dying a horrible, painful death in that rat-infested house. The patient's house was not very far from where I live, and I made the executive decision that if no one was going to rescue that poor little dog before the end of my shift, I was going round there to get it myself – even if it meant breaking and entering.

Well, fortunately it didn't come to that. After speaking to the ambulance crew in question, we found a way of contacting a neighbour, who came round with a key and took the dog in herself. What a relief – I am not going to have to resort to hustling canines in the dead of night after all.

# A Visitor to the Control Room

20 September 2006

While I was sitting at the dispatch desk, I noticed a teenage boy in a wheelchair being pushed round the call-taking area. He seemed to be having a whale of a time, his face lighting up as he took in the various screens and the photos of ambulances on the wall.

'How nice,' I thought to myself. 'I didn't realize they allowed children to visit. Perhaps it's like a modern-day *Jim'll Fix It*, or something.'

As the boy left, we all waved him goodbye.

'Who was that?' I said to Snowy, who'd just returned from her break.

'*That*,' said Snowy, 'was Banana Man with his social worker. Apparently she brought him up here to show him what we all do and teach him the implications of his hoaxing.'

'You're joking!' I exclaimed. 'That sweet innocent boy is the one who terrorized us for months? Well, if I'd known who he was I'd have given him a piece of my mind!'

'If it stops him calling, they can bring him up here every day,' said Snowy.

She had a point.

# One Chow Mein and a Cardiac Arrest, Please

25 September 2006

When an ambulance crew take a critically ill patient to hospital on blue lights, we ring the hospital to warn them. This is called (imaginatively) a 'blue call'. All the blue call numbers are programmed into our phone system, so we only have to dial a couple of digits to get them. The hospital in Romford, however, has just moved, so we have to dial the full number to put the blue call in.

T601 were bringing in a man in cardiac arrest, so I dialled the number.

Them: HELLO, CAN I HELP YOU?
Me: THIS IS LONDON AMBULANCE WITH A PRIORITY CALL.

Them: YES?
Me: T601 ARE BRINGING IN A SIXTY-YEAR-OLD MALE, SUSPENDED ...

Them: UH ... SORRY ... I THINK YOU HAVE WRONG NUMBER. THIS IS CHINESE TAKEAWAY!

I was a laughing stock for the rest of the shift. Jenny insisted on telling everyone who she spoke to, including all the ambulance crews, 'Watch out for our radio operator today ... she tried to blue a patient into the local Chinese!' Everyone thought it was hilarious. My face has never been so red!

# Communication Between
# Police and Ambulance

26 September 2006

Our computer system contains something called the 'CAD link' (CAD stands for Computer Aided Dispatch) which enables us to send calls through to the Metropolitan Police instantly, without having to speak to anyone. We can also send messages back and forth regarding each call, almost like an instant messaging service.

I had the following conversation with the police today.

Address: **PIZZA WORLD TAKEAWAY, 200 HIGH STREET, NE20.**

Diagnosis: **CALLER STATES HE IS THE KING OF ENGLAND AND WISHES TO GO TO PSYCHIATRIC HOSPITAL.**

Special instructions: **CALLER WILL WAIT INSIDE PIZZA SHOP AS HAS ORDERED A PIZZA.**

From: **LONDON AMBULANCE SERVICE**

To: **METROPOLITAN POLICE SERVICE**

Message: **PLEASE CAN WE HAVE YOUR ASSISTANCE WITH MALE PSYCHIATRIC PATIENT, POSSIBLY VIOLENT, STATING HE IS KING OF ENGLAND AND WISHING TO BE TRANSPORTED TO PSYCH UNIT.**

From: **MPS**

To: **LAS**

Message: **SORRY, NO POLICE AVAILABLE AT PRESENT. WE ARE ON CHANGEOVER.**

From: **LAS**

To: **MPS**

Message: **NO WORRIES – APPARENTLY PATIENT HAS ORDERED PIZZA WHILE HE WAITS.**

From: MPS
To: LAS
Message: NO ANCHOVIES FOR US, PLEASE.

(Twenty minutes later)

From: LAS
To: MPS
Message: PLEASE CANCEL. PATIENT HAS RUNG BACK STATING PIZZA
NOW READY. IS TAKING BUS TO LOCAL HOSPITAL.

From: MPS
To: LAS
Message: WE ARE VERY DISAPPOINTED. OFFICERS WERE HUNGRY
AND LOOKING FORWARD TO MEETING KING OF ENGLAND.

# Brenda: The End

Today we had a call from Brenda Kramer's daughter.

'Come quickly, it's my mother!' she said. 'I hadn't heard from her for a couple of days and she wouldn't answer her phone, so I've gone round and I can see her through the letter box. She's lying at the bottom of her stairs and she isn't moving! I think she's dead.'

'Oh, pull the other one,' said Jenny, who was listening to the call. 'I bet that's Brenda herself making the call again. I said an injunction wouldn't stop her.'

'She's wasting our time and the police's,' grumbled Snowy, sending a message through to the police requesting their attendance. 'I bet they put her in prison for this.'

Later, the crew told us what happened.

The police smashed the door in, but it was too late. Just as her daughter had said, Brenda was lying at the foot of the stairs, and she was dead. They think she slipped on the stairs and broke her neck. She would have died instantly, without even having time to reach for the phone. Finally, after all these years, Brenda really had been in genuine need of an ambulance.

I felt sad for Brenda. Sad that after all these years of calling us out for nothing, she couldn't have made the one call that would have saved her life. Sad that just as her new care plan had been put into place, it all turned out to be pointless. And in an odd way, I'll miss her calls, her theatrical manner, the aghast reports from the crews who attended. She was a real character.

Here's to you, Brenda.

# Where Is Sally?

1 October 2006

News of Brenda's untimely demise made me think more about Sally Wiltshire. I wish there was a way I could find out what happened to her without compromising patient confidentiality. I know her address, of course, but I can't exactly go and sit outside her house with a pair of binoculars!

I tried searching for her name on Facebook last night. Alan asked me what I was doing and, when I told him, he said I had gone mad and was getting far too attached to these crazy people I deal with at work. He doesn't understand. It's not that I am attached to the patients, I just want to know what happened to them. There is nothing worse than following a story and not knowing how it ends.

# Romance Is Dead

Alan and I have split up. I suppose it was inevitable, we've been like ships that pass in the night lately. I never understood why it was that so many people from Ambulance Control were romantically involved with fellow EMDs or paramedics, but now I understand perfectly: they are the only people who can put up with your shift work and, quite often, the only people you see regularly enough to form any kind of meaningful relationship with.

After realizing I would need to work four twelve-hour overtime shifts per month to be able to afford my own place, I have moved into a shared house with a Portuguese hippy and a gay psychiatric nurse. I've never flatshared with strangers before. Alan is staying in 'our' flat until he saves up the deposit to move elsewhere.

If I was still in my old job defluffing mice and setting up passwords, I'd probably have spent the entire weekend crawling into a bottle of vodka, stumbled into work hung-over at 10 a.m. and then spent all day playing on the Internet and eating cake in a bid to cheer myself up. No such luck here. You're not allowed an off day when people's lives are depending on you. This afternoon I took a call about a motorcycle accident. A dog had run into the road and the motorcyclist had gone straight into it. He'd come off his bike and broken his leg. The dog was killed outright. For some reason, despite the fact I deal with *people* dying every day, the thought of this poor dog being killed in such a horrible way had me welling up in tears. I had to go and take a stress break in the toilets to compose myself. And then I carried on.

# Meet Horace

6 October 2006

If there has been an increase in the 999 call rate this week, it is probably all down to one individual. Horace Halfpenny. Everyone in the room knows Horace. Every ambulance crew in London knows Horace. In fact, I wouldn't be surprised if every ambulance crew in England knows Horace. There are probably crews in Azerbaijan and Outer Mongolia who would grimace knowingly upon hearing his name. Horace Halfpenny is a homeless, alcoholic gentleman with no affiliation to any particular area. We've had him in Kennington and Kensington, in Putney and Purley, in Park Royal and the Royal Parks. There is not an area where Horace hasn't been seen. He drifts around London, occasionally stopping off at payphones to call 999. Sometimes he asks a member of the public to call for him. But the problem is always the same. *Horace's bowels are hanging out!*

Horace's bowels are indeed hanging out, but the only reason they are doing so is because of his colostomy bag, which he has a propensity to fling at paramedics, doctors and other undeserving members of the community. If he would only stop flinging the bag, the bowels would stay in. I have no idea why he keeps calling 999, because once the ambulance arrives, he verbally abuses them, sprays them in excrement, then makes off on a bus to a random location where, more often than not, he calls 999 again. On the rare occasions that he does get taken to hospital, the doctors and nurses get much the same treatment. He has been banned from at least five hospitals. Sooner or later he will be banned from *every* hospital and then God knows what he will do. Nothing ever gets done about his protruding bowels, which are quite a sight (apparently), because if he has an operation he'll just pull them out again.

Crews hate getting sent to Horace. Apparently they have taken to pre-warning dispatch: 'I'll be off the road after this call. Dirty vehicle and uniform, and filling out an LA52 for verbal abuse.'

I do not like the sound of Horace. I hope he does not take to hanging around anywhere near my house.

# Regretting my Move

My flatmates are driving me utterly insane. Anabela will not let me turn the heating on, even though it is getting so cold now that you can see your own breath. She keeps banging on about the environment and my carbon footprint. I don't give a fig about my carbon footprint, I just want to be warm enough to sleep. I went to bed in my London Ambulance Service fleece and three pairs of socks last night.

Henry is almost as bad. He borrowed my hairbrush without asking, left a pile of facial hair clippings in the sink (I hope that's what they were) and hasn't done the washing-up for a week.

To make matters worse, I hadn't been at work more than half an hour when I noticed a call on the screen from Horace Halfpenny – practically outside my house. My worst nightmare! I knew this was an unsavoury area to move to! I told the crew in no uncertain terms that they were to remove Horace from the vicinity. I do not want a colostomy bag chucked at me on my way home, thank you very much. I already have enough on my plate.

I checked back on the call later and discovered the crew had taken Horace to a hospital fifty miles away in the depths of Kent. Hopefully this is the last we will see of him for some time. Let Kent Ambulance Service clean up after him for a bit.

# Nothing to Live For

13 October 2006

I was working as a radio op on the south-east desk when a rather odd call came in. It was from a man who was doing building work on a nearby house. He heard a commotion coming from the house opposite and went to see if everyone was okay. Someone was screaming for an ambulance, but no one seemed to be calling one, so he did.

'I wonder what's going on?' I remarked to Snowy. 'I'd better listen in to the call and see if I can work it out. The call taker seems to be struggling to get any information.'

I lifted the phone and pressed the button that allows us to listen in on the 999 calls.

'Someone's not breathing!' I heard the workman say. Quickly, I sent a message down to the ambulance crew Jenny had already dispatched, to make them aware that this was a very serious call, just in case they were faffing around getting equipment on to the vehicle or something. I let them know that we'd send more information as we got it.

Before starting CPR the call taker quickly asked what had happened, in case this was a dangerous situation for our crew. The workman told him he didn't know. All he could see was a young woman lying on the floor, not breathing, with her hysterical family around her, and that the young woman was clearly pregnant. Not wanting to waste any more time, the call taker started CPR.

'I don't think we're going to find out what happened until we get there,' I said to Jenny. 'The call taker's concentrating on resus now. We'd better arrange a manager and the police.'

'Okay,' said Jenny. 'We've already got two ambulances and an FRU on the way.'

The FRU was a paramedic, the first crew were the usual technicians, but the second crew was a Green Truck, who do not usually deal with life-threatening calls. Since the second crew on a suspended is primarily there just to assist with fetching equipment, lifting the patient, looking after distraught relatives and keeping in touch with Control, and the Green Truck was far closer than the next regular ambulance, it made sense to send them. I bet they weren't expecting to see something like this when they got up for work in the morning.

The FRU arrived on the scene first, took one look at the patient and asked the workman for the phone.

'Send HEMS, please, it's a hanging!' he said.

HEMS was sent and then we didn't hear anything from any of the crews for quite some time. Jenny, concerned for their safety, decided to call the manager, who told her that everyone was still working on the patient. It had been over an hour and we wondered what was going on – had they managed to save her? Someone pointed out that if a woman dies when she is nearing full term, sometimes her baby can be saved if it is delivered by Caesarean quickly. Were they doing that?

Then the HEMS desk got a call from their doctor to say that the resus attempt had failed and that they had pronounced life extinct. The woman was too early on in pregnancy for the baby to have any chance either. One by one the crews withdrew from the scene, going off the road for that infamous cup of tea that makes everything better and prepares them to face another call – which they did, an hour later. We made sure we gave them nice calls to little old ladies for the rest of the day.

We all felt quite despondent in the control room after we'd heard from HEMS – I guess we'd all been hoping for a happy ending against the odds. We had wondered what could be so awful in that young woman's life that she had to destroy it, and her unborn child too. But perhaps the circumstances of her pregnancy were simply too dreadful to bear, and she felt it better that her child didn't have to deal with them. Or perhaps she was suffering from a psychotic illness, not thinking straight, not realizing what she was doing. You just don't know, do you? It was too horrible for words. We didn't want to think about it any more. We just pressed on, more calls, more ambulances … think about something else …

# A Day on the West

14 October 2006

Henry had a bit of a party last night, even though he knew full well I was up at 5 a.m. for an early shift. I didn't get a wink of sleep and it was still going on when I got up for work. The living room was full of saucer-eyed people with multi-coloured hair smoking funny cigarettes, and when they saw my uniform they asked if I was going to a fancy-dress party. Henry was sitting on the sofa, wearing a top with red wine spilt all down it, and drooling. He had a huge bump on his head. When I asked him what had happened, he said, 'I ran into an ambulance!' and then laughed so hard that he fell off the sofa. I didn't join in.

I was put on the west sector at work today. The west sector scares me because it has Heathrow Airport in it. I always think there is going to be a plane crash when I work there. I know that, statistically, this is not even worth worrying about, but I can't help it.

In the end there was no plane crash, but then something statistically far more likely occurred. We had a call from Horace. He is back from Kent. His bowels are still hanging out. The crew hadn't met him before and spent over an hour off the road cleaning their vehicle and uniforms and filling out a record of verbal abuse.

# What Every EMD
# Never Wants to Hear

15 October 2006

I was giving out a call to St Paul's Cray when Snowy piped up: 'Crikey! What's going on at 611 Rose Lane?'

And I sat up and stopped in my tracks. Because 611 Rose Lane used to be my address. It still is Alan's address.

'What do you mean?' I said, my heart beginning to pump faster.

'Three calls coming in, and no information on any of them!' said Snowy. 'Oh! Thirty-year-old male, hanging! I'll give it out to Orpington, shall I?'

'Let me see that!' I exclaimed, peering over Snowy's shoulder in the hope that somehow she'd got it wrong. She hadn't.

'Thanks, Orpington,' said Snowy, hanging up. She turned to me. 'What's wrong? You've gone as white as a sheet!'

'That's ...' I spluttered. 'That's where I used to live. That ... that might be Alan!'

Leaving Snowy open-mouthed, I clutched at a ray of hope and rang Alan. The phone rang out and went to answerphone. I hung up and rang down to the call taking supervisor. There were six flats in that block. Alan lived in Flat 5.

'Rosemary Jones, taking the call about the hanging,' I panted. 'Tell her – get a flat number. The block has six flats. Six flats.'

'I'm sure it's not him ...' said Snowy unconvincingly. I knew what she was thinking – while it seemed that Alan had taken the break-up well, how likely was it that there was another man in our block of his exact age who'd just undergone a suicide-invoking trauma? I felt bile rise in my throat. This was my worst nightmare, the call I'd never wanted to see on my screen.

The ticket updated.

Flat three. Flat *three*. Someone else. Not Alan.

I sat back in my seat and took a deep intake of air, feeling beads of sweat roll down my forehead as the ambulance pulled up at the scene.

A couple of minutes later my phone rang. Ignoring the strict 'no mobiles in the control room' rule, I answered it. It was Alan.

'Hello!' he said excitedly. 'Guess what! There's an ambulance, two FRUs and a police car outside! Are you at work? Did you send them? What's going on? Has someone broken their leg?'

'No,' I said. 'No one has broken their leg. You know I'm not allowed to tell you.'

'Ooh!' carried on Alan. 'Someone's crying in the corridor! I'm going to go out and look!'

'I really, really wouldn't do that if I were you,' I said. 'Look, I have to go. If Management catch me on this phone I'll be up for a disciplinary.'

The patient, my erstwhile neighbour, was beyond all help. I know this because the crew didn't convey him to hospital and they had to go off the road for a full debrief afterwards. Apparently they were a newly qualified crew and it was the first non-natural death they'd witnessed. If I hadn't found out from them, I would have found out from Alan, who sent me a gleeful text telling me they'd removed something that looked rather like a body bag from Flat 3. After due consideration, I decided not to tell him that I'd thought the victim was him, or how relieved I was when I heard it wasn't.

# How Many Ambulances Does it Take
# to Change a Light Bulb?

## 17 October 2006

Occasionally we get wildly inappropriate calls that are not your usual brand of timewaster but people who do not know where to turn and are using 999 as a kind of general helpline. I often wonder what makes them request 'ambulance' instead of 'police' or 'fire' – I guess it's just that they see the police as scary law enforcers and don't want an entire engine full of firemen turning up, so the Ambulance Service is the only option left.

One such call came in this week, at around 8 p.m. It was from a woman in her eighties who was a carer for her disabled bedbound sister, who was even older. The little old lady was very upset because the light bulb in her sister's bedroom had broken. Apparently her sister was scared of the dark, never switched the light out and suffered from panic attacks. The caller wanted to know if we could arrange someone to come round and change the light bulb. She'd pay, if necessary, she just couldn't find anyone to do it. She had no nearby relatives, no carers, her neighbours were all equally elderly, and she didn't know what to do because her sister was getting more and more distressed by the minute. The call taker, quite rightly, told the caller that she was sorry but that she couldn't help because we only deal in ambulances and not light-bulb-changing people. She recorded all the details, including the address, on a ticket, which duly popped up on our screen as an 'enquiry only'.

'Hmm,' said Jenny. 'How many ambulances have we got sitting on station at the moment?'

'Three,' I counted. 'One at Mottingham, one at Bromley and one at Greenwich.' (This is very unusual for 8 p.m – for some reason no one in south-east London fancied a trip to hospital that night.)

'And look,' said Jenny. 'There's H702 on their way back from hospital. They're going to have to drive right past this lady's house to get back to station. Suzi, could you please call them up on the radio and ask them for a mobile number so I can speak to them in private?'

I got H702's mobile number and Jenny rang the crew, who no doubt thought they were in trouble.

'Bit of an odd request here,' she began. 'How are you at changing light bulbs? Yes, light bulbs. See, we've had this call … [she explained the call] and it's just up the road. There's a couple of vehicles on station so I doubt you are about to get a call, but if you do I'll call you on this mobile number and you'll have to drop the light bulb and run.'

Jenny then rang back the old lady to tell her we had managed to find someone after all, but in future she would have to sort out a regular light bulb changer as we wouldn't do it again. Fortunately, no calls came in for that area and ten minutes later H702 were back in their vehicle, leaving behind two very satisfied customers.

'After all,' said Jenny, 'if I hadn't sent them, she would be phoning in three hours later when her sister was in the midst of a panic attack. And that would take far longer to sort out. Prevention is better than cure, that's what I say.'

# My New Flat

6 November 2006

After another sleepless night and a huge stand-up screaming row with Henry, I stormed out of the flat and went for a walk in the High Street. I happened to peer into the window of an estate agent's and saw an advert for a very familiar flat. Flat 3, 611 Rose Lane. Newly refurbished, apparently. Then I walked into the agency and asked to arrange a viewing. It was absolutely gorgeous and just about within my budget – if I work eighty hours a week for the next month to save the deposit and sixty from then on to cover the rent. I tried not to think about what happened there. After all, I bet all properties have their secrets and many must have had someone die in them. Do you know what happened to the previous owners of *your* house? If it wasn't for my job, I would never have known. I told the estate agent that I'd take it. I considered haggling the price down a little due to the potential presence of ghosts, but decided against it. I didn't want them to think I was totally macabre!

I moved into my new flat a week later, not even giving Henry, Anabela and their freezing, filthy, noisy hovel a second glance. Alan gave me a hand with my stuff. It is rather odd living in the same block as my ex, but he's leaving at the end of the month anyway and I am sure we can tolerate passing each other in the corridors until then.

I know most people wouldn't want to live in a flat knowing that the previous occupant had died a horrible, tragic death there, but strangely it just makes me feel fonder of the place. I know its secrets, I was part of the drama that happened here. I don't believe in ghosts.

That said, even I felt a little freaked out when I went into the hallway and looked up. I hadn't noticed it when I moved in, but there is a large metal pole going across the skylight. It has a discernable bend in the middle, as if, for instance, someone had tied a noose around it and then jumped.

I shall try not to look up when in the hallway in future.

# Stag-night Disaster

12 November 2006

Late on Friday night reports started to come in of a person set on fire in the toilets of the Dog and Duck pub in New Cross. At first the call takers considered that it might be a hoax or a false alarm, since (thank God!) this kind of thing isn't exactly commonplace, but this theory was quickly disproved by the fact that we took about ten calls on it, all giving the same details. Very odd, we thought. If you were going to murder someone in such a horrid and dramatic way, surely you would drag them to a field in the middle of nowhere before dousing them in petrol and igniting them? Surely doing it in a public toilet is the easiest way to get caught?

When a call like this comes in, as well as sending an ambulance, the first thing the dispatch desk does is to get on to the police and fire brigade. Most of the time they will already know because a member of the public will have called them (personally, if I saw a man on fire, my first thought would be 'fire engine!' and not 'ambulance!') but we call them anyway, to be sure they are aware and so we can coordinate our response with theirs.

The fire brigade were on their way, but they didn't have any more information than us. The police, however, were able to shed a little light on the matter. The following message appeared on screens via the electronic link.

ONE OF OUR PATROL CARS PASSED A STAG PARTY O/S THE DOG AND DUCK 30 MINS AGO. ONE MALE WAS DRESSED AS A MUMMY, WRAPPED IN TOI-LET PAPER. BELIEVE THIS MAY BE RELATED.

As the crew on the scene later reported, the police were right. The stag's friends had thought it was hilarious to dress him as a mummy and send him stumbling around outside the pub with toilet paper over his eyes. One friend thought it would be even funnier to hold a cigarette lighter to the end of the toilet paper. He had no idea how flammable the toilet paper was. Unable to stop the flames, the friends had bundled him into the toilet and tried to put them out with water. By now the man was a seething mass of flames and had caught the attention of the other pubgoers, which was when we were called.

By the time our ambulance and HEMS team reached the patient, the fire was out, but he had 40 per cent burns and was blue-lighted into hospital in a critical condition.

I think it's safe to say that the wedding is off.

# One of Those Nights ...

15 November 2006

You know it's going to be one of those nights when you've only been in work for half an hour and you've spent at least 50 per cent of that time trying to explain to a woman who has caught her finger in a child's pushchair why she isn't going to get an ambulance any time soon. The conversation went a little like this.

Woman: SO YOU'RE SAYING, UNLESS I HAVE A LIFE–THREATENING EMERGENCY, I HAVE TO WAIT AGES?
Me: ER ... YES.

Woman: BUT I MIGHT HAVE BROKEN A FINGER!
Me: YES, AND THAT ISN'T A LIFE–THREATENING EMERGENCY.

Woman: YOU'RE TELLING ME THAT IF YOU BROKE YOUR FINGER, YOU WOULDN'T CALL AN AMBULANCE?
Me: I CERTAINLY WOULD NOT. I WOULD CALL A TAXI, IF ANYTHING. CAN'T YOU CALL A TAXI?

Woman: I CAN'T AFFORD A TAXI! I AM NOT A MONEY TREE!
Me: HOW ARE YOU GOING TO GET BACK FROM THE HOSPITAL?

Woman: WELL, I'LL CALL A TAXI!
Me: SO WHY CAN'T YOU CALL ONE NOW?

Woman: BECAUSE ... ARE YOU BEING SARCASTIC WITH ME? YOU ARE SO RUDE!
Me: I AM NOT BEING RUDE. I AM MERELY POINTING OUT THAT IF YOU CAN'T AFFORD TO GET TO THE HOSPITAL, YOU CAN'T AFFORD TO GET BACK EITHER, AND YOU WILL BE STUCK THERE.

**Woman: BUT ... BUT ... LISTEN, YOU ... THERE'S A CHILD HERE!**

**Me: ER, I SEE. AND IS THE CHILD HURT OR ILL IN ANY WAY?**

**Woman: (PUTS PHONE DOWN IN FURY.) ...**

Well, that call remained at the bottom of the pile for the next half-hour, until another call came in – a cancellation from the woman's neighbour. She said that she had given them a thorough telling off for misusing the Ambulance Service and then lent them a tenner to get a taxi to the hospital.

I must remember that for every idiot who is rude and/or misuses the service, there is another, like this lady's neighbour, who is kind and sensible and who has the ability to restore my faith in human nature.

# Sally Mystery Solved

16 November 2006

Yesterday we received a call in the dead of night from an address about two miles from where we last saw Sally. It was from a 26-year-old female, suicidal, threatening to put razor blades into her vagina. The landline she was calling from was registered to a 'M Wiltshire'. Sally's surname, different initial. Could this be Sally, staying with a relative? How many 26-year-olds are there in north London with that surname and a penchant for inserting razor blades into delicate orifices?

As soon as the call taker hung up, I knew I had to call back to see if it really was Sally.

The young woman on the other end of the phone was in a terrible state. Hyperventilating, crying, talking gibberish.

'It's the Ambulance Service,' I said. 'Help is on the way – I just need to take your name. For our records.'

No answer. I wasn't even sure she was listening to me. 'Oh God, oh bloody hell,' she moaned. 'I can't take it any more, I just want to die ...'

The ambulance and police crew were just pulling up. I tried once more. 'What's your name?'

'Sally ... Sally Wiltshire ...'

And the line went dead.

I almost got up and punched the air in jubilation that Sally wasn't dead.

Sally was taken to hospital later. She was covered in slash marks on her arms and legs and had indeed cut her own vagina with a razor blade. It wasn't the first time she'd done this and I suspect it won't be the last. My happiness that she was still alive was dented slightly – I'd wanted the reason Sally had stopped calling to be because she was better. And maybe she is getting better – after all, she had gone nine months without calling, whereas for a while she'd been calling almost every night. Perhaps it's just baby steps. Good luck, Sally. I wish she could know that we are all glad she is alive and hoping she recovers.

# The Art of Understatement

20 November 2006

We got the call as '25-year-old female injured ankle playing football'. We sent a Green Truck. It took half an hour to arrive, merrily trundling along to the football pitch without a blue light in sight or a siren to be heard. No one with the patient called back to enquire where it was during the time it took to arrive.

When the Green Truck did arrive, they immediately called for assistance. It was an ankle injury alright. The woman's foot was hanging by a thread, pointing in an impossible direction, and the sharp ends of two broken bones were sticking out through her sock. The sort of injury that really turns my stomach. Five minutes later a paramedic crew arrived, dosed the patient up with a large amount of morphine, splinted the leg and blued her into hospital.

When the crew asked why no one had mentioned how bad it was on the phone, or had called back during the half-hour they were waiting, they said: 'Well, we wouldn't have called if it wasn't serious, and we didn't call back because we knew we'd be a low priority – no one dies of a broken leg, do they?'

They had a point, of course, but in view of the large number of people who *would* call for a simple sprain or knock, we had assumed – due to the lack of evidence to the contrary – that it was just a minor injury. They, meanwhile, had assumed we'd know it was serious by virtue of the fact they'd called 999, and that a serious fracture was one of the *least* serious things we get called out for. And if people used the Ambulance Service correctly, they would have been completely right. The fact that so many people make inappropriate calls makes it hard for us to identify people who are in genuine need, and to respond appropriately.

# What Am I Going to Say?

25 November 2006

I was listening in to one of the suspended calls on our desk the other night. It was from a man who had found his elderly mother dead. It appeared to be too late for CPR. All he kept saying was: 'I told my sister not to visit Mum today because she was too poorly. I told her to come tomorrow. What am I going to say to her?'

# Happy Ending

30 November 2006

Two bobbies on the beat were perusing their local area when they saw a black taxi pulled over on the side of the road, with the driver slumped over the wheel. They sprinted over, prised open the taxi door and saw that the driver was not breathing.

One policeman dialled 999 directly on his mobile phone. Usually the police radio their control room if they need an ambulance, but going direct can save a few vital seconds. The other policeman pulled the patient from the taxi and placed him flat on his back at the side of the road. Having established that the patient was definitely not breathing, he had already begun CPR by the time his colleague had given the location to our call taker. The call taker thus had an easy job – he just had to check with the first policeman that the second was doing it correctly (he was) and stay on line to keep us updated.

As I'm writing this, it occurs to me that the number of times I have tried to give CPR instructions and had them refused because the caller already knows how to do it is so minimal that I can count it on the fingers of ... well, one finger, actually.

The ambulances (two of them, and an FRU for good measure) were on the scene within five minutes, and then we heard nothing, until I got the blue call on the radio.

As I've mentioned before, if someone is not breathing for longer than three minutes and not receiving CPR, they will most likely die or be brain damaged.

'This is T103, blue to King George's with a 60-year-old male, post cardiac arrest, was in VF, one shock given ... now pulse 90, BP 130/88, respiratory rate 12 ... be there in 8, over ...'

(Non-jargon translation: 'His heart wasn't beating, but we zapped him with an electric shock thingy and it started again, and now he's probably healthier than half the patients that get blue-lighted in.')

I felt a little bit like replying to the blue call with: 'Woo, T103! You got him back! Fancy that, eh? Big pat on the back!' but of course that is not professional and would interfere with notifying the hospital, so I didn't. However, if 'T103' are reading this, I can say 'Well done!' now, and also a big 'Well done!' to those two policemen, without whom the patient would certainly have died.

It is, sadly, quite rare for us to get a call when a patient is brought back after cardiac arrest. Often crews blue them in while still trying to resuscitate them, and often they are unofficially pronounced dead at the scene. So when we get a blue call like this, there's a little celebration on the dispatch desk, and we all feel happy for a few minutes and do a little dance around the table, until the monitor shows that there's another call coming in, and then we all go back to work and forget all about it.

# The Worst Kind of Call

1 December 2006

What's worse than a suspended call? A suspended call that involves a young person. These are far less common than you'd think. As far as I can recall, I have taken eleven such calls in nearly two and a half years.

The call which popped up on our screen this morning was another. It simply read '21-year-old male suspended'. We immediately dispatched two crews but, not wanting to send them into a dangerous situation, Jenny lifted the receiver and listened in to the call. She could hear a hysterical woman describing a horrible scene.

The patient was her flatmate. She'd got up that morning to go to university, knowing he had to be up at the same time. When she'd finished her breakfast and he still wasn't up, she went and knocked on his door. He hadn't answered. She'd peeked her head around the door to see if he was there. He was. Lying in the bed, eyes open, his face purple, stiff, cold, obviously dead. The caller had screamed her head off, then grabbed the phone and continued to scream down it. The call taker was gently trying to persuade her to take a closer look and start CPR, but the caller was having none of it. She wouldn't even touch him. I couldn't blame her – I wasn't even there and I could tell this patient was beyond any help.

At this point a man – another flatmate, I think – took the phone. He was calmer, but confirmed what I suspected: when the call taker asked him to start CPR he said there was no point, the patient was clearly dead. The call taker asked him if he knew what had happened, and the caller said he had no idea. The patient was epileptic, but he hadn't had a fit in ages, and otherwise he was perfectly healthy. He just couldn't believe what had happened ...

The crew arrived at this point. It was less than ten minutes before they called back to say yes, the patient was 'purple plus' and could we arrange for the police to attend due to the patient's young age. There were no obvious suspicious circumstances, he said. In fact, there was no obvious cause at all, and it seemed likely the patient had simply had a fit in his sleep, causing his tongue to block his airway and rendering him unable to breathe.

I could still hear the patient's flatmate wailing in the background.

This incident was a wake-up call to all of us about how deadly fits can be. We get hundreds of such calls every day, and 99 per cent of the time, these are routine – the patient starts to recover before we've even got off the phone and doesn't always need to go to hospital. This was a reminder to us that if the patient doesn't have someone to turn them on their side and check their breathing afterwards, a fit can be anything but routine.

# Have I Hurt Someone?

## 2 December 2006

At about 4 p.m. we were called to a road traffic accident – a woman pushing a pram hit by a large car. We had at least ten calls from the scene, with some of the callers incredibly distressed. The call takers managed to piece together what had happened – while the woman had been thrown to one side as the car had hit her, the pram had been caught under the wheels of the car. The car had carried on until it hit a wall and the pram, with baby inside, was completely crushed and inaccessible. Another woman, who was later identified as the baby's mother, plunged towards the wreckage and hopelessly tried to get the baby out. The woman who'd been hit turned out to be the baby's grandmother, and the mother had only avoided being hit because she was walking a few paces ahead.

According to witnesses, the driver of the car, a middle-aged woman, staggered out and, with a glazed expression, asked the passers-by why everyone was screaming. Had she hurt someone?

The fire brigade arrived and cut the baby out, and the crew rushed his crushed body to the hospital. It was just a formality, there was nothing they could do to save the baby. He was too badly injured. The crew were so upset by the call that they went off the road for a good couple of hours afterwards, and here in Control, we felt a bit off the road too. What an awful thing for the crew to deal with, and what about the other victims? There was the poor grandmother lying injured in the road as the pram was snatched out of her hands and crumpled, and the mother witnessing the whole thing, only steps away from being close enough to help.

Half an hour later we got a call from the local police station. They wanted an ambulance for a fifty-year-old woman in custody, who'd taken an overdose. 'Please note,' said the special instructions, 'this is the driver from the earlier incident in Long Way.' That was why she'd crashed into the wall. She'd taken an overdose of painkillers with alcohol and then, realizing what she'd done, she'd decided to drive to the hospital to get help. Ironically, she hadn't called an ambulance because 'she didn't want to waste their time'.

The crew, who worked at the same station as the original crew (who were still off the road recuperating from their ordeal), knew all about the incident. When I told them who their patient was, you could almost hear them wince. But it's an ambulance crew's duty to treat all their patients with respect, no matter who they are or what they've done.

The gang of relatives, friends and witnesses who'd gathered outside the police station had no such compunction. They shouted and swore and threw stones at the ambulance doors as it sped off to hospital.

# Feeling Chilli

3 December 2006

**Caller:** I'VE GOT A CHILLI IN MY VAGINA!

**Call taker:** UM. OKAY. WHAT'S THE ADDRESS WE'RE COMING TO?

**Caller:** NO ... I JUST WANTED SOME ADVICE.

(We're not actually allowed to give advice over the phone, but on this occasion my colleague thought this was less like advice and more like Stating the Bleeding Obvious ...)

**Call taker:** WELL, MY ADVICE IS TO TAKE THE CHILLI OUT OF YOUR VAGINA. AND SOME MORE GOOD ADVICE IS NOT TO PUT CHILLIES IN YOUR VAGINA. THEY ARE FAR BETTER IN CURRIES.

**Caller:** THANK YOU!

**Call taker:** (FIRING UP THE PSYCHIATRIC CARD JUST IN CASE.) ARE YOU SURE YOU DON'T NEED AN AMBULANCE?

# Keeping it Together

'What on earth is going on here?' said Snowy, pointing at the screen. 'The diagnosis is "baby not breathing" but the call taker has marked that the call is delayed as he doesn't know the location of the patient. All we have is the location that the call has come in from.'

No sooner had she spoken than the call taker ran over to explain what was going on. The call had come from a neighbour. The couple from the upstairs flat were running around hysterically shouting that their baby was not breathing. The neighbour had gone straight inside to call the ambulance and, after giving the details to the call taker, ran back to get them to bring the baby in and start CPR. But when he went back into the corridor, he found that they were gone. He went back and told this to the call taker, who urged him to go and look for them and bring them straight back.

'How stupid can you get!' said Jenny, as she sent an ambulance out. 'Suzi, please do a general broadcast telling all crews in the Bromley area to be on the look-out for a couple with a sick baby. They can't have gone far.'

The ambulance, which wasn't far away, was just pulling up at the location when we got another call from a nearby main road.

'Big Long Road, Bromley. (Caller unable to be more specific.) Couple seen standing by roadside with baby, looking distressed, baby appears unwell. Caller not on the scene. Was driving past.'

(You have to love these callers who judge a situation serious enough to call an ambulance but not to actually stop and help these poor people in case it makes them five minutes late for work ...)

I got back on the radio and told the ambulance crew to head back to the main road. At that moment one of the FRUs called.

'This is SE46 – I think I've got your suspended baby. Report to follow, over.' Then he disappeared, presumably to start work on the baby, while I told the ambulance crew exactly where to find him.

Half an hour later the crew blued the baby, who was indeed in cardiac arrest, into hospital, and the FRU rang to tell us what had happened.

'I'd just heard your GB as I was heading down Harrow Road. There they were, a crying couple getting into a black cab, asking to go to the hospital. The cab driver, thankfully, had some sense and was refusing to take them. He was just dialling 999 on his mobile when he spotted me and waved me down. By then the mother had climbed into the back of the cab and was hysterically insisting he drive them to the hospital, two miles away. The father was trying to wrestle the phone from the cab driver and shouting: "Just drive!" I don't think they even realized I was a paramedic. The baby was completely blue and lifeless. No one was doing CPR. I got into the back of the taxi and I had to practically drag them out. It was only then that I started resuscitation.'

I worked out that there must have been ten minutes between the initial call from the neighbour and the FRU paramedic starting CPR. Ten minutes without breathing or CPR means almost certain death or severe brain damage. Less than three minutes means a significant chance of recovery. The original ambulance had arrived on the scene at the location of the call in three minutes precisely. If only they'd kept their heads and stayed put, the baby would have had a chance …

It would be heartless to blame these parents for the death of their child – and, for all I know, he may have been beyond help from the start – but no one can say he was given the best possible chance. The parents, obviously, 'lost it'. They panicked. They thought to take the child to hospital, but not much else. They didn't listen to the neighbour or the cab driver, both of whom knew that an ambulance and CPR would be needed to give the baby any chance of survival. Their panic and inability to keep it together failed their child.

# Weeping Willows

5 December 2006

The call on our screen was from Greater Manchester Ambulance Service, and there was a lot of detail crammed into a short space.

'30yof? "mental breakdown". Has just had daughter taken away from her. ? suicidal. Sister in Manchester concerned for her safety. Sent text saying "goodbye". Patient's name Anna, sister's name Jessica.'

A lot of the time, we get calls like this, turn up, find the patient drowning their sorrows but otherwise okay and make a reassuring call to the concerned relative. Other times, we find the house locked, with no answer at the door, call the police round with their enforcers to break it down ... just at the point the 'patient' returns from shopping. Such patients are rarely impressed.

On this occasion, however, the ambulance crew found the door wide open, and the flat empty. It was night-time and the ambulance crew called me on the radio to ask what they should do next. I called Jessica, the sister, to explain what we'd found.

'She's gone somewhere to kill herself!' sobbed Jessica.

'Do you have any idea where?' I asked.

'No,' said Jessica. 'I don't know London at all! She's only been living there two months. She moved there to get away from her partner when they split up, and took her seven-year-old daughter with her. But they said her daughter's got to stay with her partner. They came and took her today. She's not coping at all, she's gone crazy. I seriously think she's going to do something stupid ...'

'Do you have her phone number?' I asked.

'Yes,' sniffed Jessica, 'but it's no good, she won't answer.'

I took the number anyway. Sometimes people *will* answer when it's a number they don't recognize, even when they're ignoring their family and friends. Even in the depths of their suicidal impulses, curiosity wins over. Sure enough, the phone was picked up on the second ring.

'Hellooo?' said a wild, tearful and somewhat drunk-sounding voice.

'Is that Anna?' I said. 'This is the Ambulance Service. We've had a call from your sister, Jessica. She's very concerned about you, and she'd like an ambulance to check you over. Can you tell me where you are so we can do that?'

'I don't WANT an ambulance,' wailed Anna. 'I just want to go to sleep! I am nothing but trouble to everyone. I'll be wasting their time. There are people there who deserve help! Don't waste your time on me when people are really sick! Tell them to go away!'

We can't force anyone to have an ambulance if they don't want to, but there's no rule against gently trying to persuade them to change their mind, and I certainly thought Anna could do with talking to someone.

'Anna,' I said, 'you're not wasting anyone's time. We're here to help people like you. Your sister has called us, we can't let her down. I'm not allowed to let the ambulance leave until they've seen you and made sure you are okay.' (This isn't strictly true but I was pretty sure she wouldn't know that.)

'I'm not okay, I'll never be okay,' said Anna. 'I just want to go to sleep. I'm very tired.' Her voice was slurred and distant.

'Have you taken something?' I asked, a feeling of dread rising.

'Tramadol, zopiclone ... I took them all ... I just want to go to sleep ...' she muttered.

Oh, great. I've spent enough time on the phone to the poisons information hotline, investigating overdoses for crews, to know that this was a potentially fatal overdose. We needed to find Anna.

'Where are you?' I asked. 'We need to find you. Please tell me where you are.'

'It's a nice place to go to sleep,' rambled Anna, seemingly missing the point of my question. 'There's grass, and a weeping willow. I like weeping willows.'

'Where's this weeping willow?' I asked. 'Is it in a park? Are you near your house? The ambulance crew are at your house. Can you go back there?'

'I won't go back there if they are there,' said Anna. 'Goddamn it ... I left my travel card there, now I can't go back for it ... still, it's okay here, under the weeping willow in the park ...'

You see what she was doing? With one breath, she was telling me she didn't want to be found, with the next, she was giving me clues. She was in a park with a weeping willow, and she'd not had her travel card with her, so she must be walking distance from home.

'Anna,' I said, 'please let us help you. You've taken an overdose which is most likely going to kill you if you don't get to hospital quickly. You're not going to go to sleep, you're going to die and if you die you'll leave your sister devastated and you'll never see your child again. Is that what you really want?'

'No! I just want to sleep! I just want the pain to end.'

'We can help you. Just tell us where you are.'

'I told you! Under the weeping willow!'

And with that, the line went dead. I tried to call back, but she wouldn't answer. Seemingly, she was challenging us. She was giving us enough information to work out where she was, but not making it easy for us. We'd have to show that we really wanted to find her by putting some detective work in. I turned my attention back to the radio.

'SE22. I've just spent ten minutes on the line to your patient. She's taken an overdose of tramadol and zopiclone and she's in a park, walking distance from her address, sitting under a weeping willow. I don't suppose you have any idea where that might be?'

'Oh, the weeping willow!' said SE22 sardonically. 'Right! I reckon there must be about five hundred weeping willows in Greenwich. We'll start looking, but this could take some time. Perhaps you'd better notify the police, over.'

Funnily enough, at that exact moment a new ticket came in from the police: 'Uphill Park, SE10. Under weeping willow tree. 30yof. ? psychiatric, crying hysterically, talking to self.'

I directed SE22 to the park and crossed my fingers. Just because we knew where she was, it didn't mean we'd find her. After all, it's easy to hide in a park in the middle of the night if you don't want to be found.

Five minutes after SE22 arrived at the park, they had Anna on board and were on the way to hospital. I guess she didn't try too hard to hide. I guess she did want to be found after all.

# Collapse Behind Locked Doors

## 8 December 2006

One of the ambulance crews rang in for help today.

'We're outside an elderly woman's house,' they told me. 'Her district nurse called us because she's come to change her dressings but isn't getting any answer at the door. Apparently she's prone to falls. Before the police kick the door in, can you just check that she's not already in hospital? Her name is Mrs Hilda Turnip and her date of birth is 8 August 1929.'

'Sure thing,' I said. 'I'll call you back.'

First I checked the call logs to see if we'd received any calls to that address in the last few days. Nothing. Then I rang the closest hospital, the Princess Royal, who confirmed she was a patient there, but hadn't been in since her operation three weeks ago. I tried the second-closest hospital, Lewisham, but they'd never heard of her. Just to be thorough, I tried King's College too – they have the nearest specialist cardiac care department, so if she'd had a heart attack she might have gone there. But she wasn't there.

I rang the crew back.

'No luck,' I said. 'Tell the police to get that enforcer out.'

'Right,' said the crew. 'Thanks for trying.'

Half an hour later the crew were back on the phone.

'We're, um, not going to be conveying, but we have been delayed on scene. I thought I'd better let you know,' the crew told me sheepishly. 'It turns out that Hilda hadn't collapsed at all. She'd forgotten her appointment with the district nurse and gone shopping at Somerfield. When she got back and found the door off its hinges, she assumed she had been burgled, and when she heard voices, she thought she'd caught the burglars in action. As one of the policemen came to the front door, she whacked him with her umbrella! Fortunately, she's only a little old dear, so she didn't do too much harm, but we're just cleaning up his cut and making sure he is okay.'

# What Did You Do This Weekend?

9 December 2006

One of the worst things about this job is having to work at weekends. I'm always acutely aware of the things I could be doing when, instead, I am rising at 5 a.m. to go and sit in a stuffy control room, wearing green and talking to idiots, timewasters and the occasional critically ill person. My general procedure for working Saturdays is to sit with a glum look on my face, moaning: 'The football will be kicking off about now ... and now my friends will be in the pub ... and now they'll be out clubbing ... and POOR ME!'

And then sometimes, something happens to make you stop feeling sorry for yourself, and to remind you that there are much worse places you could be.

An ordinary family, consisting of a man and a woman in their late twenties and their ten-month-old son, who apparently were not similarly cursed with weekend working, were on a busy single-carriageway A road on the outskirts of our patch. Perhaps they were returning from a picnic in the forest or a day by the beach. Dad was driving and Mum was sitting in the back seat with baby on her lap.

Going the other way on the road was a black taxi.

Who knows what happened to make the family's car career into the path of the taxi? Perhaps baby grabbed at Dad's hair, causing him to momentarily lose concentration. Perhaps Dad was distracted by the football results. Maybe he swerved to avoid a squirrel. Whatever it was, it was enough to make the two vehicles meet head on when both were travelling at 70 mph. The taxi driver was jerked viciously in his seat, hitting his head against the steering wheel and slumping forward, semi-conscious. Mum crunched into the seat in front of her, and felt a crack in her spine followed by the contrast of the numbness in her legs and the agonizing pain of her splintered arm. The unsecured baby, meanwhile, flew unimpeded into the front of the car, smashing his head against the windscreen, shattering the glass and collapsing in a bloody heap on the bonnet, just in front of his shell-shocked father.

Before the FRU paramedic even touched the patients he phoned control for urgent back-up. Three ambulances, preferably paramedic crews, and the helicopter, please. Unfortunately, the helicopter was out, so a Delta Alpha was sent instead – that is, an on-call HEMS doctor from their home address in a blue-light car. The FRU reported that the baby had a GCS of 3 (GCS stands for Glasgow Coma Scale and is a measure of consciousness – 3 is the lowest possible score), that he had a head injury and that one pupil was completely blown (indicative of brain damage).

Three ambulances arrived on the scene, their blue lights flashing and sirens blaring. Over the next hour, three ambulances left the scene, one by one.

The first ambulance contained the baby. He was now in cardiac arrest. The massive head injury he'd suffered had proved too much, and there was nothing anyone could do. Perhaps the only reason he was taken to hospital, rather than being pronounced dead at the scene, was to show the parents that everything that could be done was being done.

The second ambulance contained the taxi driver. With a serious, possibly life-threatening head injury, he had little idea of what was going on, which was perhaps a blessing in disguise.

The final ambulance to leave the scene contained Mum and Dad. Of course, they weren't anyone's mum and dad any more, but they didn't know that yet. Mum also had very little idea of what was happening. Collared and boarded, all she knew was that her body didn't feel right, that pain was everywhere and her baby was not with her.

Seated in the same ambulance, clutching a compress to a dripping wound on his head, watching the paramedics work on his wife, silent, in disbelief, was Dad. He was conscious and alert and not in any real pain. He'd been the lucky one – the only person to escape from the crash without life-threatening injuries. Yet his life would be ruined by this family day out just as much as if he had been the one who died.

# Allocator Training

I got to work this morning and headed for the radio operator's chair as usual.

'No, not there,' said Jenny. 'You're sitting here.' And she gestured at the allocator's seat.

'I can't sit there!' I panicked. 'That's the scary seat!'

Since I've been working on the dispatch desks, I've always wanted to have a go at allocating. I've watched Jenny intently, trying to pick up what she was doing, and I've practised in my head, making decisions about calls and seeing if they match up with hers. Actually becoming an allocator would be such an honour but also a big, terrifying step. Once you're allocating, you're in charge of the desk. Other EMDs come to you for advice and you are expected to make your own decisions without help. You're supposed to know what you're doing. And while I do think I know what I'm doing, I always have the safety net of being one of the more junior staff on the desk and therefore having someone to look up to.

'Suzi, it's 7 a.m. on a Sunday morning,' said Jenny. 'There's absolutely nothing going on. You'll be fine. Come on.'

I sat gingerly in the seat and stared at the blank blue screen.

And stared, and stared. For five minutes not a single call popped up.

'Oh, this is simple!' I said. 'What a breeze! I wish I'd done it earli – Aargh! A call on my screen!'

'Yes, a call – just like the thousands of other calls that we've dealt with while you've been working on this desk. What are you going to do with it?'

'Asthma in Orpington! Well, I'll ring St Paul's Cray and give it out. Hello, Cray? Who's out first for an asthma attack? Number Three? Coming down!'

There, I did it.

As the day went on the desk became busier and busier. Leg injury in Lewisham? Ring Lee. Breathless in Bexley? That's one for Barnehurst. Car crash in Catford? Forest, you're next. There, I'm an old hand. Pass me a big sign with ALLOCATOR written on it. Simple.

Of course, it didn't stay simple. By midday there were more calls than there were ambulances. It was time to start making decisions.

I looked at the screen. There were two Cat A calls and one available ambulance. One call had been waiting longer, but the other was closer to the ambulance. I looked at the diagnoses. One was an eighty-year-old with breathing problems. The other was a thirty-year-old with a sore neck and throat and fever ... tonsillitis or meningitis? I sent an ambulance to the old lady and got Snowy to broadcast the other one. No ambulance offered up. I started to panic at the red call sitting on the screen. It appeared to be angrily glaring at me, turning redder by the minute. I turned to Jenny.

'Help, I'm holding a red call! It might be meningitis! I'm going to kill someone!'

'It's fine. Someone will come up in a minute. You've only been holding it thirty seconds. This happens every day, remember?'

'Not on *my* screen, it doesn't!'

'Look, there's L319 come up at the hospital. Send them the call!'

I breathed a sigh of relief as the screen went blank again. L319 got to the call within the required eight minutes and did not blue in the patient, so it seemed it was tonsillitis after all.

By the end of the day I found I was juggling several calls: holding some for CTA and Green Trucks, ringing people to advise a delay, shouting over to other desks to borrow their ambulances, putting crews on breaks and giving instructions, and all without making a total idiot of myself or having a mental breakdown.

The allocator's phone rang about half past six. It was someone from the Hazardous Area Response Team.

'Can I speak to the senior on the south-east please?'

I was about to pass it to Jenny, when I remembered and said, 'Yes, that's me.'

# More Allocating

I'm learning more and more about allocating as I go on. It's all simple when there are more ambulances than calls, but the real skill comes into play when you have several calls and have to decide which call gets your only available ambulance.

There are several factors I have to take into consideration. The most important is the priority of the call – we're supposed to reach red calls within eight minutes and amber calls within nineteen minutes. Of course, the point of having a human allocating rather than doing it all by computer is that we can look at what the call taker has written and realize that while two calls may have the same computer-assigned priority, one is clearly more likely to be life-threatening than another. The next factor is how long the call has been waiting, so I'll send on calls of the same priority in roughly the order they came in. How far the ambulance is from the call is also important. For inner-city calls I rarely send ambulances more than a mile or two. In the suburbs three and a half miles is acceptable, and on the outskirts of London it can sometimes be as much as seven miles. Any further than that can mean you are upsetting the distribution of ambulances throughout your area, and another closer ambulance is likely to pop up before the one you sent from miles away arrives on the scene – or another call will be received in the area you sent the ambulance from. Also, accidents are more likely to happen when ambulances are driving miles on blue lights – and we try to fix accidents, not create them!

We have to make sure that calls get the right type of ambulance. Some of our ambulances are manned by paramedics and some are manned by technicians. A paramedic is basically the same as a technician, but there are a few extra procedures they can do and some more drugs they can give. We must send a paramedic if the patient is fitting, giving birth, dying or in severe pain. There are also different types of vehicles – the older vehicles won't take a patient in a wheelchair, for example, and their trolley beds won't carry very obese patients.

It is very tempting to send ambulances to the calls where the callers were polite and helpful before you send to the ones where they swore at the call taker and hung up the phone, but you can't do this.

Really, allocating is just like playing a computer game, such as Tetris. If you make the right decisions, the calls will disappear from your screen and you will have plenty of ambulances to play with. If you make the wrong decisions, the calls will stack up and fill your entire screen. Of course, unlike Tetris, you can't just give up when the calls are coming at you too fast. You have to find a way to fit the calls and ambulances together somehow. The satisfaction of giving out your last call is immense. The empty screen is my favourite sight.

# Allocating Decisions

I had a difficult decision today while allocating. I needed to ask Jenny for reassurance that I'd handled it right – but of course I can't keep asking her for ever!

At about midday I was holding two calls: a Fitting (amber) and an Old Woman Fallen, On Floor, Leg Injury (green). K701 became available near Fitting, and seconds later K702 became available near Old Woman. But K702 were a paramedic crew and K701 weren't. Fitting might have needed a paramedic crew, and Old Woman probably didn't. I had three options – send both ambulances to the calls they were near and ask K701 to tell me if they needed another vehicle with paramedics or not, send both to the fitting (so as to get the patient both a quick response and the paramedic they were likely to need), or send the K702 to Fitting and K701 to Old Woman, meaning both calls got the most appropriate response, but not the quickest response.

I went with the last option, which unfortunately meant the crews passed each other on the dual carriageway. One of the paramedics from K702 rang up to grumble about my decision, but I explained to him my thought processes and he seemed to understand. I didn't add that it was my first week of allocating and that I was a nervous wreck, so please do not challenge me!

Afterwards Jenny said that I held my ground well and that sometimes with allocating there are no right or wrong answers. You just have to be able to make a decision which you can explain and stick to. She added that I should not enter into debates with crews about my decisions either. We would not tell them how to treat their patients and they should not be telling us how to allocate ambulances!

The scariest thing about allocating is that you are responsible for any decisions that you make and, while there are guidelines and protocols for most things, they don't cover every eventuality. And anyway, if a patient dies, it won't be much consolation to their family if you stand up and say, 'But I was just following protocol!' The consequence of this is that I feel terribly anxious until I get every single call off my screen, and I treat every call as if it were a national emergency, even if it's obviously a load of rubbish. I'm told this feeling passes after a while.

# Dreams

I'm actually having dreams about allocating. Sometimes I am trying to give calls out but all the details are in Greek and I can't understand them. Sometimes I'm looking for an available ambulance but they have all disappeared or gone to south London. Sometimes I realize a cardiac arrest has been sitting on my screen for half an hour and I haven't covered it. I wake up in a blind panic. And the first thing I think when I wake up is, 'Oh God, I fell asleep, what about all the calls?' Then I realize I am actually at home.

# Suicide

For some reason, it seems the depressives of London have all decided to pick the same weekend to attempt to end it all. Even the nurses answering the blue call phones at the hospital have commented on the number of overdoses and slit wrists that are coming in. I'm told that it's a myth that more people commit suicide in the run-up to Christmas – apparently the most common month to take your own life is May, though no study ever seems to have come up with a concrete reason why this is so – but it certainly feels that way to us. Perhaps more people attempt suicide in December and call 999 as a result – or maybe it just feels that way because Christmas is supposed to be a happy time, when everyone is having fun, and those who do not fit the mould stick in the memory.

There was one call that stood out, though. A woman in her thirties. Her husband had just walked out, leaving her with a selection of children aged between four and twenty-one. Beside herself, she couldn't go on. Then and there, in the presence of her kids, she'd decided to commit suicide. You may ask yourself what sort of woman would kill herself in front of her children, but if you want proof that the balance of her mind was disturbed, look no further than the method she used to die.

She drank hydrochloric acid.

If you're not familiar with hydrochloric acid, it's a pungent, fuming corrosive that will burn through almost anything it comes into contact with. It is highly reactive and dangerous. Just inhaling it can be fatal because of the damage it will cause to the lungs. It is used for removing rust from metals, unblocking drains and in oil production for dissolving rock. The acid burned through one of the paramedics' gloves and ruined the ambulance's blanket. It took nearly an hour for the crew to clean up the vehicle afterwards.

The patient's children tried to help her and, in doing so, got the chemical on their bodies, causing some nasty burns, so the crew took them in too. A blue call was placed, and the patient was semi-conscious and breathing at the time but, as the crew told me later, they didn't think she could possibly survive. That acid would eat her up from the inside out.

On the way to the hospital the patient's ten-year-old son told the paramedic that, as soon as he was back from the hospital, he was going to kill himself too.

# Horace Again

21 December 2006

Horace is back on our sector. Just in time for Christmas. I got a call from the police last night, saying they'd found an intoxicated male lying by the side of the road with 'what appeared to be a very serious abdominal injury'. I just had a feeling about it. I sent a message back to the police, telling them that we were on our way and asking them what the patient's name was.

'Mr Halfpenny,' came the reply.

I just knew it!

I felt really apologetic as I called the crew on the radio to let them know what they were going to. I could almost feel their faces slump.

'Not again!' said one of them. 'We went to him last week! I reckon there should be a Horace rota and that you shouldn't have to go to him more than once in a month. It should be the law! Can you make a note that we're going off the road to clean up after this?'

'Certainly,' I said. 'Sorry to do it to you.'

True to their word, the crew went off the road an hour later.

'Horace was on fine form today,' huffed one of the crew. 'He got in the vehicle, tried to assault my crewmate – "tried" is the operative word, he missed and fell over, and only succeeded in spilling beer and the contents of his colostomy bag all over the trolley bed. We took him to the hospital, where he went mad in A&E and threatened to shoot the consultant if he didn't get him a drink. The consultant called security and now he's banned from the hospital. We're under strict instructions not to take him to that hospital ever again.'

'Like any other hospital wants him!' I tutted. 'Well, thanks for letting me know. I had a feeling something like that would happen. Take as long as you like to clean up.'

No sooner had I put the phone down than Jenny groaned.

'I don't believe it!' she exclaimed. 'Horace is calling in again! From outside the hospital! Right, that's it. Get the police running and I will send a manager down there. We need to sort this man out. Perhaps we can arrange for the crew to take him to Australia and dump him in the Outback this time?'

'He'd be back within the week,' I shuddered.

When Jenny rang the manager, he happened to be with the crew who'd just been to Horace. Much to our surprise, they actively wanted to go back to him. Their vehicle was still dirty, but they didn't care as he would only dirty it again anyway. I think it had become a point of principle with them, and they were as eager to see the back of Horace as I was.

Everyone did their best. The manager apparently gave Horace a lecture about misuse of the service, backed up by the police, and the crew told him there was no way he was ever setting foot in their ambulance again.

Horace knew when he was defeated, and shuffled off – beer in hand – on to a double-decker bus headed for Edmonton Green.

I broke the bad news to the north-east allocator.

# Tragedy

Tragedies are common in this job. Ambulances aren't supposed to go to happy events. But usually, in every call, there's a glimmer of hope, a small positive that we can take home from the situation. Occasionally this is not so. Occasionally a job is just horror from beginning to end and makes you shudder and feel cold inside.

To begin with, there was no indication that the call was anything out of the ordinary. Just before Christmas, a 37-year-old female, in labour. Waters broken. Baby due on New Year's Day. How sweet. Sixteen-year-old son making the call. Panicking a bit. As we sent the ambulance, we rolled our eyes and made the usual comments about maternataxis and how after sixteen years as a mother one should know how to get to hospital by taxi and ...

The ticket updated to indicate that the pregnant woman was having a fit. Okay, we ate our words and realized this was a medical emergency. We made sure the crew knew that – although, of course, that wouldn't make them drive there any faster, would it? An emergency call is an emergency call!

Just as the ambulance was pulling up, the ticket updated again. It now read: '37yof in labour, waters broken. EDD 1/1/07. Now ? Fitting now. ? cardiac arrest.'

We weren't sure what was going on and there was a suspicion amongst us that the teenage son was either giving the wrong answers to questions – as a result of panicking, or a language barrier – or, as sometimes happens, the mother was deliberately making the situation sound worse than it was to get an ambulance more quickly. After all, it's quite a leap from being in labour to being dead, and the two states are not easily confused. While we naturally have these thoughts, we never act on them. Never doubt the integrity of the caller, as they taught us in training school. A second ambulance was sent to assist straight away.

Half an hour later the blue call came. 'It's H702, blue to hospital, with a 37-year-old female, full-term pregnancy, in cardiac arrest. We'll be five minutes.'

So it *was* as bad as it sounded. The desk went very quiet, wondering what on earth had happened.

An hour or so later we spoke to the crew, who were having a cure-all cup of tea back at station.

'They delivered the baby by emergency Caesarean,' one of them told us, 'but he was already dead. They managed to get an output from the mother, but as they were taking her up to Intensive Care, she arrested again, and this time they couldn't get her back.'

'How awful,' I said. 'What happened?'

I thought he'd say that she'd suffered from eclampsia or a pulmonary embolism – something big and deadly that no one could have prevented.

'She choked,' said H702. 'On a fish bone. She was in early labour and she was having something to eat with her kids before she went to hospital. As she ate, she collapsed. Her son, who made the call, didn't realize what was wrong. We only found out as we tried to intubate her. There it was, blocking her airway. We got it out, but by that time she'd already been down too long.'

So that was it. Something as simple as a fish bone had ended two lives, robbed a family of their mother and the baby brother due to be born on New Year's Day. Instead of welcoming the new arrival, they'd be planning a double funeral.

It's calls like this that make you appreciate the fragility of life and the knife edge that we all live on.

# Nasty RTA

While offices all over the world are steadily winding down for Christmas, Ambulance Control just gets busier and busier. The cold weather has a negative effect on the elderly, and festive drinking does little for the young. Staffing levels are not great because everyone's off with the flu, and the overall result is Too Many Calls, Not Enough Ambulances. I was just about managing to keep on top of it by getting poor Snowy to lose her voice broadcasting the calls we were holding and cajoling the long-suffering ambulances to turn around a little bit faster at hospital.

Then the call which was to be the final straw came in. A car had hit a motorcyclist on a busy, fast road right in the middle of my patch. The car actually drove over the top of the motorcyclist before it managed to stop. He had serious head and chest injuries. About twenty calls came in at once from panicked bystanders and, as is the way with bystanders, only about half of them had the address right and only half of them knew what had happened (some said a pedestrian had been hit by a car, some said a motorcyclist had fallen off his bike, some just knew a man was lying in the middle of the road), resulting in a spattering of similar-sounding calls around the area. The danger in situations like these is that one might assume they are all the same call, when really there have been two similar incidents in the area, so three ambulances were started while the call takers managed to ascertain that there really was only one incident. One ambulance was then cancelled. I kept two running because the general consensus was that the person was unconscious, and two callers seemed to think he was also not breathing. Unfortunately, HEMS could not be dispatched because it was coincidentally dealing with another call on my patch (a child who'd fallen down concrete steps and sustained a serious head injury with a GCS of 3 – i.e. completely unconscious) but the HEMS team in the control room spoke to the crew to give them advice over the phone.

The advice of the HEMS team was to get the patient to the Royal London Hospital as quickly as possible. This is the hospital the helicopter operates from, and it has advanced trauma care and a neurology department. The crew were just heading off when they hit a stumbling block – the patient had come round and was what we call 'cerebrally irritated' – in other words, his head injury made him confused and violent and he was lashing out at the crew who were trying to help him. There were already three paramedics/technicians on the back of the ambulance, but they were unable to restrain him. They radioed for urgent police assistance and another crew. These were all sent straight away, along with the duty manager. So there were now:

Five paramedics/technicians in the back of the ambulance treating the patient.

One driving the ambulance.

An unknown number of police officers restraining the patient.

A manager making sure the crew were okay.

An FRU still at the scene of the accident, checking over the bystanders and the car driver, and babysitting all the empty vehicles.

I am not even sure how all those people managed to fit in the back of the ambulance. They decided to take him to the local A&E to get his condition stabilized, rather than make the long trip to the Royal London. (The local A&E most probably organized another ambulance transfer to the Royal London for specialist care later.)

So that was it for the ambulance cover on my patch. My calls were mounting up – I had a call waiting for a 33-year-old male in cardiac arrest and had absolutely nothing to send to it. My neck was saved by a very kind offer from a crew who had actually finished their shift and were taking the vehicle back to station, but who offered up for some impromptu overtime. In the end the patient was beyond any help, but it's not a chance you want to be taking.

I was so stressed when I left the building, I thought my head was going to explode.

# Christmas Night Shift

26 December 2006

Ugh! What a horrible shift! Last year we were on days for Christmas, and we had a party kind of atmosphere in the control room – people wandering in and out of the room with plates of food and everyone falling asleep in front of the mess room telly during their breaks, while a steady trickle of (mostly rubbish) calls came in. Steve came up to the room with a bunch of mince pies, and we all had fun with a raffle and a Secret Santa.

Well, what a contrast. This year staffing levels both on the road and in the room were at an all-time low. The call rate, however, was relentless. I don't know what it is about Christmas these days. When I was a child (growing up in a suburban, middle-class, almost exclusively Christian area) absolutely *nothing* was open and it was unheard of for people to do anything other than sit and eat turkey and play board games with their family. These days it's all different – as I made my way to work, I noticed shops and pubs open in every street, and even one open hairdresser's! Those shops and pubs were later full of fights and stabbings and people generally not full of festive cheer. There was not one Christmas Comedy incident such as 'choking on mince pie' or 'impaled on Christmas tree', which was very disappointing. There was instead a steady trickle of green calls (because of the lack of public transport and increased taxi fares), a whole bunch of chest pains (indigestion, anyone?), plenty of Domestic Incidents and a couple of rather sad cases, such as a woman whose sister, far away in Scotland, had taken an overdose alone in her flat, and a homeless lady who had rung for an ambulance in the hope that it would take her to a hostel in central London so she would not have to spend Christmas night on the streets.

We felt sorry for her, but not sorry enough to send the ambulance ten miles out of its area when we had a screenful of sick and injured people waiting.

But there was one call that was worse than all of them. It came early in the shift and managed to ruin our moods before we'd even begun. A middle-aged couple went to visit their son on Christmas afternoon. Getting no answer at the door, they'd tried his mobile phone again and again, rung round his friends and knocked and knocked. As the hours went by they'd become more and more worried until eventually the father had had enough. Convinced something terrible had happened, he kicked the door in.

His wife let out a scream. There, in the doorway, dangling from the banisters, was a pair of legs. The father dropped the presents he was carrying in horror. Their son had hanged himself, on Christmas Day.

# A Thank-you Letter

29 December 2006

Management handed us a Christmas card with a picture of a jolly robin on it today. In it was the following letter.

Dear South-east Desk

I am writing to thank you for the patience and politeness you have shown to my sister Sally, who is a regular user of your service. Sally has serious mental health issues and must be difficult to deal with sometimes. She was sexually abused as a child by our uncle and this has had a devastating effect on her. Because of her drinking, we as a family found it hard to cope with her. Our parents blamed each other and consequently split up, and Sally's problems got worse. She went into foster care and I lost touch with her for five years. This year we got back in touch and Sally has come to live with me. I have tried to support her the best I can, but I have little experience of supporting people with mental health issues and it is hard to keep your cool when your drunken sister is waving razor blades at you.

Recently I had to call you when Sally had slashed her own neck. She was nearly unconscious and had lost so much blood that I thought she'd bleed to death in my arms. Your call taker was amazing and really helped to calm me down and give me instructions on how to help Sally until the ambulance arrived. Fortunately, she pulled through. I'm pleased to say she was sectioned after that and is now in rehab for her alcohol problems.

The hospital has arranged for us to have family counselling sessions once she has completed rehab, and Sally seems to be quite receptive to this idea. They've also been taking her to the dentist to have her teeth fixed and this has raised her morale no end. There was a time when I almost hoped I would find she had passed away in her sleep, just so her suffering would be over, but now I am starting to hope we are finally turning the corner.

Once again, thank you to you and all your colleagues,

Matthew Wiltshire (brother of Sally Wiltshire)

2007

# My Mother's Accident

3 January 2007

I had a phone call from my mother today. She has broken her wrist! It was the dog's fault. She (the dog, not my mother) insisted on being taken for a walk in the middle of the night and then decided to climb one of the steep banks outside my mother's house. My mother is never firm with the dog. I would personally say: 'Kipsy, no. Stick to the path or there's no walk at all.' So they went up the bank, and my mother, who is almost a pensioner, slipped over and broke her wrist.

I once told my mother that ambulances do not like being called out for injured wrists, and she took this a bit more literally than I intended, and drove to the hospital, which is ten miles away, using one hand! This was not quite what I had in mind. I meant get a taxi! Or ask someone else to drive you! Driving with a broken wrist is the sort of thing that causes road traffic accidents – which, of course, ambulance crews do not mind being called out to at all.

I despair.

# A Call Outside the Hospital

The only unusual thing about the call was its location. The patient, a middle-aged woman suffering from chest pains, was a passenger in a car, about 100 metres from the local hospital.

'That's stupid,' said Jenny. 'Why didn't they just keep driving to the hospital? The nearest ambulance is further away than the hospital. By the time it reaches them, they could have been there.'

Still, the rule is that if someone wants an ambulance, they get one. If they want one for someone with chest pains, they get one as soon as humanly possible.

The ambulance crew that we sent, however, were able to shed some light on the matter. The caller had provided us with the patient's name, and they recognized it.

'We just saw these people leave the A&E!' they told me. 'They were having a barney with the receptionist as we got there. The patient didn't have chest pains *then* – she'd accidentally taken double her dose of iron tablets and wanted to be checked out. A&E is busy at the moment, and they were told it was a four-hour wait, which they weren't happy with. At that point they saw us coming in with our last patient. We'd blued her in with a severe asthma attack, so of course she went straight in. Seeing that, they announced that they'd go out to the end of the road and call an ambulance because then they'd get seen straight away. The receptionist told her that it didn't matter how they arrived at hospital, how quickly they were seen depended on what was wrong with them. Clearly they realize that people with chest pains get priority. You couldn't give them a call back and let them know we're on to them? This seems like a blatant abuse of the service.'

I agreed, but obviously I couldn't go ringing back the caller and throwing accusations at them. I had to tread carefully.

'This is the Ambulance Service,' I began. 'I just need a little more information for our crew. I believe you were in A&E a little while ago, is that correct? Could you tell me what the outcome was?'

'I, er ...' said the caller, who was the driver of the car and the son of the patient. 'No, we weren't there. That was my brother. He, er, went on ahead. And then he came back and told me that A&E had told us to ring 999.'

'The ambulance is further away than the hospital,' I said truthfully. 'You would get there faster if you carried on driving.'

You are not allowed to tell someone that they ought to make their own way to hospital, but there is no rule against providing them with facts that might encourage them to do so.

In the following three minutes, I had a frustrating conversation with the caller in which he contradicted himself several times and talked a large amount of nonsense in an attempt to convince me that he really needed an ambulance. I ran out of time. The crew pulled up behind the car. I sighed. I knew these people were lying, but the crew would have to take her at her word and treat her as a suspected heart attack and do all the necessary checks. What a waste of time! I was sure that they'd find nothing wrong, so the patient still wouldn't be seen straight away, but because she was alleging chest pains, she'd take precedence over some of the other patients in A&E who'd been waiting longer.

The crew had only been on scene for a couple of minutes when they radioed for urgent police help.

'Urgent! Police, please! This man has just accused me of assaulting him, and I didn't lay a finger on him ... and now he's going for my crewmate!'

I felt awful and bumbled something on the radio about how I'd tried to call them back as I dialled the police. The crew didn't care, of course – they just wanted the police to turn up and save them.

The police were on the scene in a couple of minutes and I arranged for the duty manager to meet the crew back at the station.

I held my head in my hands. As Control staff I feel a responsibility to keep the crews on my sector safe. It's we who make the decisions about what situations to send them into, and whether they need the police with them. I felt I should have somehow picked up on the phone that these people were potentially violent – although, really, they gave no indication that they were anything other than pointless timewasters.

As soon as the crew were back, I rang them and apologized profusely, explaining that I'd been on the phone to the caller at the time the ambulance had arrived.

'Don't be silly, it isn't your fault,' said one of them. 'I think Tim and I were just so wound up by what we'd been sent on that we confronted them straight away. One of the sons took exception and said that if we didn't get his mother seen immediately, he'd report us – for assaulting him. He was about ten feet away at the time! Then he started pushing us around. Fortunately, at the sound of the police sirens, they all scarpered. The police got their number plate, though.'

'Can you describe the car?' I said. 'I'd better warn other crews if we any get similar calls tonight.'

'It was a red Zafira,' said the crew, 'but don't worry too much – we think they've left the area. Their parting shot was that they were taking the patient to Queen's Hospital instead.'

I was rather amused to note that Queen's A&E was partly shut due to overcrowding that night. I hope they had an even longer wait there.

# Horace's Demise

This morning we received a call from the fire brigade attending a blaze in a council tower block. The report came in from the first paramedic on the scene: 'We need HEMS – we've an adult male with 50 per cent burns. He's close to cardiac arrest.'

'How awful,' said Snowy. 'That poor man. I hate calls like this.'

Later, the manager gave Control a call to let us know what had happened. The patient was still alive, but they weren't optimistic about his chances. He'd been taken straight to hospital by helicopter – meaning that the priority was to save his life, rather than get him to a burns unit to treat the burns. He also let us know the patient's name.

It was Horace Halfpenny. It turned out that he had only recently been housed by the Council after years of homelessness. And somehow, he'd managed to set fire to that home. Now it seemed that – just like Brenda Kramer – Horace was going to die. As much as Horace is a pain in the neck, I did feel sad. I wanted him to stop calling because he'd learnt his lesson, not because he was dead. Like all our regulars, he was an institution. The silence of London's phone boxes will be noted.

How tragic that he had died just as he found somewhere permanent to live.

# FRU Assaulted

10 January 2007

This week the south-east desk acquired a bunch of FRUs. There have always been FRUs in the south-east, of course, but previously they were run by their own desk. While we could see what they were doing, we didn't have any control over them. The FRU desk is gradually closing down, and the FRUs will soon be entirely controlled by the same people who control ordinary ambulances. So far, I've much preferred having them on the desk – it's more work but makes things easier in the long run.

However, our first weekend with the FRUs on the desk was marred by a horrible incident. We got a call to a 'man lying in the road'. In 99 per cent of cases the 'patient' turns out to be someone drunk, or a homeless person sleeping. Members of the public are reluctant to investigate, in case the patient is a dangerous lunatic, but what they forget is that ambulance crews are just people too and are just as likely to get hurt by a dangerous lunatic. Because most of these patients are harmless, we usually leave it up to the crews to decide whether they want police assistance. On this occasion, they were happy to go and assess the patient without the police.

An FRU emergency medical technician named Fred was first on the scene. He spotted the patient straight away, opened the door of his car and took his equipment out. Fred knew the patient wasn't dead when the man got to his feet and raised his fist. Fred didn't even have time to reach for his phone to ring for help before he fell to the ground. The man didn't stop then – he carried on kicking and punching Fred while he was on the ground. Fred felt everything go black ...

Minutes later, Jim and Bob arrived on the scene in their ambulance. They saw the man lying on the ground too, and Fred's car, but there was no sign of Fred. Then Jim looked a little closer and saw that the man lying on the ground *was* Fred, barely conscious and covered in blood. Bob jumped on to the radio and pressed his priority button to alert us.

'This is K606. We need urgent police assistance! SE66 has been seriously assaulted, we've just found him lying in the road, covered in blood. My crewmate is assessing him now and I'll get back to you on the radio.'

Horrified, we called the police and got another crew and a manager down to the scene straight away. We all felt a bit guilty – from the safety of the control room we'd sent poor Fred out to this call and let him be assaulted. Perhaps we should have called the police or only sent a two-man ambulance? But that's easy to say with hindsight – you simply don't know which calls are going to turn out to be dangerous, and hundreds of calls like this one pass without event every single day. Our guilt then turned to anger – what kind of revolting low-down scumbag punches and kicks a paramedic as he tries to help them? What a disgusting, repugnant excuse for a human being. I hope he gets run over by a runaway ambulance and gets taken to the grottiest hospital in London with *two broken legs*! People like that make me sick.

It was also the worst assault I have ever seen on an ambulance crew and I wondered to myself if it was worse because Fred was on his own – would the 'patient' have dared attack *two* paramedics in the same way? Are solo responders really a good idea, especially at night in 'dodgy' areas? You don't see police officers going around on their own, do you? The principle of having FRUs often gets a lot of stick because they are seen as a way of meeting response-time targets rather than delivering the best patient care, and this incident has certainly done nothing to persuade me that we should have more of them.

Jim and Bob blued Fred into the local hospital because of his head injury and possible loss of consciousness, but we were later told that there was no serious injury and that he was being allowed home today.

Get well soon, Fred.

# He's Back

15 January 2007

So, in the week since Horace Halfpenny's house fire, the phone booths of London have been quiet. There have been no more calls to people whose bowels are hanging out. Colostomy bags have remained unflung. Ambulance crews everywhere have breathed sad sighs of relief.

Then, tonight, a call from a phone box.

'My bowels are hanging out!' exclaimed Horace. '*And* I've got 50 per cent burns!'

# Fingers Crossed

20 January 2007

I have applied for an allocator position. After slaving over a hot application form, writing a load of nonsense about how wonderful I am, for four whole night shifts, I got the good news today that I am through to the next stage: a written assessment paper. If I pass that, then it's an interview with Management. If I pass that, then it's new epaulettes and more money – with the responsibility for making Important Decisions resting firmly on my shoulders.

# Teamwork and the Disaster Desk

23 January 2007

It's become a bit of a running joke that whenever I work on a particular desk on the other side of the room, everything kicks off and there is calamity and disaster. Well, the other week I worked on that particular desk as an allocator, and it was the day from hell. There were three open-leg fractures, an old lady crushed by a milk float, a stabbing, a bottling, a fight between forty people, and an extremely suspicious death ... but one call overshadowed the rest.

The Desk of Disaster, unlike my usual home (the south-east), contains large patches of countryside – the no-man's-land between London's suburbs and the territory of the neighbouring ambulance service. Even on blue lights, running from the nearest ambulance station, it takes at least fifteen minutes to reach these areas. Of course, not a lot tends to happen in these areas, so they don't generally cause much concern, and we now have Active Area Cover – getting the ambulances to drive around the local area while making sure they are spread out. (This is every crew's favourite – they hate it because they'd rather be in a nice warm ambulance station, and who can blame them?) We have an ambulance hovering around the one village in this area anyway, which meant when we had a call to an eighty-year-old man who had fallen and banged his head, we were on the scene within five minutes. Super!

Unfortunately, fifteen minutes later, another call came in from the same rural place, and now the nearest available ambulance was eight miles away. It was at one of those big posh country houses up a track, miles from the main road. Response-time hell. I gritted my teeth and silently prayed it was going to be something trivial, because we had nothing for it.

'Toddler fell in swimming pool,' typed the call taker. 'Not breathing.'

Now, I don't panic. This job requires one to have a clear head and an unflappable nature at all times. But if I was going to panic, that would have been a good moment for it. You may just have seen a bead of sweat on my forehead if you looked closely. There I was, using my fledgling allocating skills on an unfamiliar desk, working with people I'd never worked with before, and I had a suspended toddler in Outer Mongolia that I couldn't cover! This was not good.

The first thing I did was to dispatch that ambulance eight miles away in suburbia. I can imagine their faces as they saw the address and diagnosis, but they didn't question it and started running on the call straight away. The second thing was to stop the radio op, who was in the middle of dealing with something else, in her tracks and demand that she broadcast the call straight away. (First rule of dispatch manners: don't interrupt the radio op, it is very rude and irritating. Second rule of dispatch manners: when you have a suspended child, drop everything, including manners.) A crew at the nearest hospital heard the broadcast and offered up straight away. They were still five miles away, but a three-mile improvement. I sent them and cancelled the first crew. We were getting there. Checking the log, I saw an FRU had been dispatched from three miles away and HEMS had also been sent (these are handled separately by other desks in the same room).

Then our prayers were answered. The crew who'd been on Active Area Cover in the rural area, and who were just leaving for hospital with the elderly gentleman on board, called up to tell us they would attend the call to render aid to the child until the others arrived. (They later explained that they'd had a third person, a student paramedic, on board, who sat with the elderly man while they dealt with the child.) They were less than two miles away.

Meanwhile, as my colleagues on the Disaster Desk and I performed the less urgent tasks such as notifying the police, the DSO (ambulance crews' manager) and our managers, two call takers were on the phone to people at the scene. Both these call takers did fantastically and afterwards the crews rang up to ask us to pass on their thanks. One call taker was speaking to an adult male at the scene and got us the full address and directions very quickly. The other was speaking to the true heroine of the story – a teenage girl who was at the poolside. It was this girl who'd spotted the toddler in the pool and dived in to drag her out, and now, with the call taker's instructions, she was performing perfect CPR, which she continued doing right up until the moment the first professionals arrived.

It's a bit strange in the control room when you get a complicated call like this, because there is so much to do until the crew arrives on the scene. But once they get there, it all goes quiet and there's nothing you can do except wait – oh yes, and deal with the stream of calls for heart attacks, road traffic accidents and teenagers with flu that have come up in the meantime.

About an hour or two later we had a call from the DSO, who let us know the latest. It was very tentative good news – the toddler had been taken to the Royal London by HEMS and was alive, but in a very serious condition. All the crews involved were going off the road for a stiff cup of tea (except the crew with the old man on board, who had to stop at the hospital to drop him off). HEMS told us that the toddler was on a ventilator and was undergoing tests on her brain. They'd let me know the outcome next time I was in.

I thought this was a pretty good example of teamwork and how well we can pull together when we've got a genuine emergency on our hands. If one piece of the jigsaw – the professionalism of the call takers, the quick thinking of the crew with the old man on board, the prompt action of the crew at the hospital, the heroism of the teenage girl on the scene, the way we on the Disaster Desk coordinated everything – had been missing, the child would have been dead before anyone arrived on the scene. It just goes to show that, while we might all bicker about each other (lazy crews that spend too long at the hospital, unsympathetic Control staff who bully crews that have done nothing wrong, call takers who can't spell, unhelpful members of the public, etc.) when it really counts, none of that matters.

I'd like to say there was a happy ending to the story, but this isn't *Casualty*, and there wasn't. Two days later, when I came in for my next shift, HEMS told me that the tests on the toddler's brain had come back with bad news, and she'd subsequently died. The only consolation was that her organs had been suitable for donation – which they wouldn't have been if she'd died before she got to hospital – and so, even though our efforts didn't save her life, they indirectly saved others.

# Itchy

25 January 2007

Last night a woman called us to complain that she had had an itchy vagina for two months, and then promptly switched off the phone. This means that we were obliged to send an ambulance to her, since there was no way of contacting her to tell her that we weren't.

Once there were absolutely no outstanding calls of any nature within ten miles of our sector, I rang the nearest ambulance station, explained the situation and apologized. Fortunately, I got a male paramedic with a sense of humour.

'That's alright, love! My crewmate and I will go and take a good look! 'Ere, Jon, you'll never guess what we've got!'

# The Percy Pig Incident

26 January 2007

It was the middle of a boring, quiet midweek night shift and one of our crews requested a service run to a nearby twenty-four-hour garage. (A service run is when an ambulance leaves its normal area to run an errand of some variety. They are still available for calls.)

'No wonder they want to go to that one,' Snowy remarked. 'It's got a Marks & Spencer's Simply Food! I bet they're after Percy Pigs.' (Percy Pigs are a Marks & Spencer own-brand pig-shaped fruit-flavoured sweet rather popular with bored EMDs doing night shifts.)

'I want some Percy Pigs!' I complained.

'So do I!' said Snowy, rubbing her empty stomach.

'G602, your request for a run to the fuel station is granted,' I said over the radio. 'But only if you pick us up some Percy Pigs while you're there. Over.'

We all giggled at the joke – mainly the fact I'd said 'Percy Pigs' over the air.

A bit later on in the night, the same crew requested a service run to headquarters to 'drop off some important admin'. We agreed – it wasn't busy and we had plenty of cover in our sector.

'What important admin can a south-east crew possibly want to do at Waterloo at four o'clock in the morning?' grumbled Management.

Fifteen minutes later the crew marched into the control room and placed two huge bags of Percy Pigs on our desk! We couldn't believe it! We'd only been joking, but they had actually bought us the sweets and driven halfway across London to deliver them! I love ambulance crews sometimes!

Five minutes after they arrived, before we'd even had a chance to thank them (or share the Pigs with them), the central desk received a call to a cardiac arrest just down the road from Control. Fortunately, G602's Pig Run had put them in exactly the right place to reach the call quickly, and off they went. The patient was blued into hospital, and if he lives, it'll be entirely down to those Percy Pigs.

# A Waste of Time

We received a call from a young man who'd accidentally cut his arm on a railing. According to him, there was uncontrollable bleeding, so it was an amber call. The crew raced to the location he'd given us – 'outside number 1, Lavender Gardens' – only to find absolutely no one there.

'This is K801,' the crew told me on the radio. 'Number 1, Lavender Gardens is a newsagent's, there is no one outside. We went inside and the shopkeeper hasn't seen anyone. Can you give it a call back, please?'

I called the origin back.

'We're outside the address you gave, and you're not there ...' I said.

'I am there,' the patient told me. I noticed he didn't sound at all worried or distressed – as you might imagine someone who'd called for an emergency ambulance would be. I checked with the crew, who double-checked with the shopkeeper that they were outside 1 Lavender Gardens.

I went back to the patient. 'You are definitely not outside number 1, Lavender Gardens,' I said.

There then followed a long conversation which was largely gibberish and which, on the whole, gave me the impression that this patient did not know where he was, who he was, or what an ambulance looked like. Getting the crew to do several orbits of the area yielded no information either. There was no sign of any patient anywhere.

The ambulance crew, growing impatient, started bellowing in my ear, asking if they could give up yet. As I was still on line with the caller, I sent a message to their MDT explaining that the caller didn't really know where he was and that I was trying to find a suitable meeting point.

'I've an idea!' piped K801 on the radio. 'Tell him to meet us at Queen – Elizabeth – Hospital!'

I spluttered with laughter out loud, momentarily forgetting that I still had the phone in my hand. Fortunately, the caller was engaged in asking a passer-by for directions and didn't hear me. He was apparently having difficulty understanding the word 'junction' and the fact that the first house he saw in the road was not necessarily number one. Oh, and apparently he wasn't even in Lavender Gardens.

Meanwhile, K801 had also lost patience and informed me they were going to circle the streets, making as much noise as possible, and that I should inform them if I heard sirens in the background of my phone call.

Thirty seconds later: *NEE NAW NEE NAW NEE NAW!*

'K801 – STOP! – over!' I bellowed into the radio. Mission accomplished. Patient found.

It was less than ten minutes before I heard from K801 again.

'This rather odd young chap had a minuscule scratch on his arm. He'd called us out for a plaster. Strangely enough, we don't stock plasters. I offered him a vacuum splint or a sling but he wasn't interested. Luckily, I was able to point him in the direction of the newsagent's that he'd called us to in the first place, so he's gone to buy his own, and now we're available again. Over.'

# Allocator Assessment

The assessment went well. I knew the official answer to 'How many ambulances do you send to a plane crash?' (six) and the truthful answer (however many you have available, which will be fewer than six, so you broadcast it on the radio and then all the crews finish with their patients as quickly as possible and head down there, whether you like it or not). I knew the station codes for every ambulance station from Tolworth to Chase Farm. I knew what form a crew needs to fill out if Horace Halfpenny throws his colostomy bag at them yet again, and I knew only too well that an LA60 is a Lateness Report Form.

I didn't know the call sign of the Command Control Vehicle at Waterloo, but neither did any of the other potential allocators. Nor did any of the five members of Management I asked, or any of the paramedics at Waterloo Ambulance Station. The general consensus was that this was a stupidly obscure question and, if none of the above people knew the answer, it really couldn't be that important.

# Baby Stabbed

4 February 2007

It was about 10 p.m. on Friday night, and we had a call to a stabbing. Sadly, there is nothing unusual about this at all. What was unusual was what the call taker wrote on the ticket next – the age of the patient. Sixteen ... sixteen *months*.

'That can't be right!' I thought and, as soon as I'd dispatched the ambulance and called the police, I picked up the phone to listen in to the call. Instantly, I recoiled from the cacophony that greeted me. A woman was crying hysterically down the phone. A man was shouting in the background. Another woman was shrieking. Some other, calmer voices could be heard in the distance, but I couldn't make them out. The only thing I couldn't hear was a baby.

'Is the baby conscious?' asked the call taker. So it *was* a baby! What on earth had happened?

'Yes!' shrieked the caller, moving away from the phone to shout something in a foreign language at one of the people in the background.

'Is the baby breathing?' continued the call taker. 'Hello, hello? I said, is the baby breathing?'

'Yes!' said the caller.

The call taker was evidently having the same thought that I was: if the baby was conscious and breathing and had just been stabbed, why couldn't we hear him? We all know that some callers – especially those in a panic and those who do not have English as their first language – just answer 'yes' to everything, thinking they will somehow get the ambulance faster by answering all the questions more quickly, irrespective of whether they give the correct answer or even understand the questions in the first place.

'Is the baby alive?' said the call taker. 'Is the baby dead or alive?' It sounded brutal, but it was totally the right thing to say. If the baby wasn't breathing, we needed to know.

'Baby alive!' said the caller, amongst a lot of hollering and flailing that was mostly not in English and was totally incomprehensible to me. The call taker in question is one of the best, and she pressed on admirably, trying to get more details of what had happened and to get the caller to perform first aid – but, really, it was like banging your head against a brick wall. There was no way this woman was ever going to calm down.

I put the phone down. I still hadn't heard the baby cry.

Seconds later a second call came in for the same address. It was being made by the infinitely calmer, English-speaking neighbours, who'd been alerted by the fracas. They were able to explain what exactly had happened. Apparently, in the midst of an argument between the baby's mother and father, the mother had grabbed a knife and lunged at the father, who was holding the baby. The neighbour didn't know whether the father or the baby had been the intended target. I wondered to myself if anyone could stab a sixteen-month-old – rather a large target – by accident, and considered the possibility that the mother had stabbed the baby to spite the father. Even if the father was the target, the crime is only marginally better. Who could stab their husband as he holds their child? I can only assume the mother was mentally ill but, even so, you can only allow for so much. Such a horrid, violent crime against her own flesh and blood – a baby too young to defend himself and too young to have done anything to deserve it – made my skin crawl.

HEMS were good enough to keep us updated on the baby's condition. He was alive, and he only started to cry when the HEMS paramedic took him from his father's arms. He was rushed to hospital and operated on straight away. Although HEMS said his injuries were life-threatening, I assume he survived, because we'd have heard about it on the news by now if he hadn't.

# Are You Sure?

7 February 2007

My allocator interview was on Monday.

On the whole, I thought I gave a good account of myself. I knew lots of important and obscure stuff (including the call sign of the CCV at Waterloo, which I eventually found in a training manual) and I talked all the jargon that is important to Management and made sure my name badge was on display and that my uniform was neatly ironed.

And then Management asked me a really simple question. I am not allowed to reproduce the actual questions asked in my interview – and it probably wouldn't mean a lot to you anyway – but suffice to say that if you had asked me this question on my first week at training school, I would have known the answer. In fact, let's just pretend the question was 'What noise does an ambulance siren make?'

'Naw nee,' I said.

'Are you sure?' said Management.

'Absolutely certain,' I said. 'Naw nee.'

'Are you sure? Do you want to think about that?' he urged.

'Aha,' I thought. 'They are trying to catch me out here, they are testing my confidence in my answer. Well, I will not be fooled. It's *naw nee*.'

Of course, once they said, 'No, it's not, it's *nee naw*,' I realized what I'd said and that of course it wasn't 'naw nee' and that I'd even answered the very same question correctly in the assessment. I went back to the control room kicking myself and telling everyone who would listen what a total moron I was. They were never going to give me the job now. I'd blown it.

This afternoon, Management came to the control room and

summoned us out, one by one, like the Grim Reaper. Some hopeful faces returned crestfallen. Then it was my turn. I was taken to the major incident room and asked to sit down. I grimaced and prepared myself for the bad news.

'Well done, Suzi. You have been successful!' he said.

My jaw actually dropped. My mouth formed a big round 'O' and my eyeballs nearly popped out. I couldn't speak. I was not expecting that.

'Are you sure?' I eventually said.

I cannot remember what happened next so I hope it was not important. The next thing I knew I was back in the control room, sitting at my desk, trying not to jump up and down with excitement, and suddenly there was a call to a person under a train. Oh my God, I thought, I can't handle this right now. And then, of course, I did.

Because I am an allocator now!

# No One Died of a Broken Leg

10 February 2007

We got a call from a local rugby pitch with a substantial – perhaps rather too substantial – amount of graphic detail: 'Rugby player has split leg open, bone protruding, foot pointing in wrong direction.' Yuck! My worst nightmare! It's at times like this I am grateful I am the one sending the ambulance and not the one who has to witness such things. And now I'm an allocator and likely to be staying in the control room for the rest of my life, the closest I'll ever come to seeing one is on a football match on TV!

I sent the nearest available ambulance without delay.

Three-quarters of an hour later, the crew placed a blue call. Although blue calls are usually for patients whose lives are in immediate danger, and people tend not to die from a broken leg, a serious injury like this can result in amputation. It needs surgery as soon as possible, as well as specialized trauma doctors, so the blue call helps the hospital to prepare.

It was literally seconds after the crew had given the blue call that we received a further call from the rugby club.

'Second patient,' it read. 'Forty-year-old male has fainted.'

'Ha, ha, ha,' I laughed, 'these rugby players aren't as hard as they look. I bet he took one look at that fella's leg and came over all funny. Quite frankly, I don't blame him. So would I.'

Then I stopped laughing. The call taker had updated the call.

'Patient has stopped breathing. CPR in progress.'

'Snowy, quick, GB this for someone closer while I send a Greenwich crew from station.' Greenwich was four miles away – we really needed someone closer than that.

'General broadcast all mobiles on channel 1, currently holding a Cat A call for Woolwich Rugby Club, a forty-year-old male in cardiac arrest ...'

'*Ding, ding, ding!*' went the radio as two nearby crews offered to help. I cancelled the Greenwich crew and waited.

'*Ding!*' went the radio again. This time it was the crew who were blueing in the patient with the broken leg.

'We're going back to the rugby club,' they told Snowy. 'Could you advise the hospital that we're delayed bringing our blue call in? We were on our way but our patient heard your GB and insisted we turn back.'

'All received,' said Snowy. 'There are two vehicles on the way to the rugby club, please render aid until they arrive and then I'll show you continuing with your blue call.'

I felt so sorry for the guy with the broken leg. Imagine sitting in the back of an ambulance, in excruciating pain, worrying about whether you are going to lose a leg, thinking that things couldn't get any worse, then hearing that one of your friends has just dropped dead – possibly due to the stress of seeing your injury occur!

Half an hour later, all three ambulances were at the hospital. The guy with the broken leg went straight into his surgery. As he went under the anaesthetic, the doctors crowded around his friend, pumping his chest, injecting him with drugs, attaching monitors, shocking him with the defibrillator. But there was nothing they could do. By the time the first patient woke up with a steel pin in his leg, the doctors working on his friend had called time of death, covered his face and taken the body to the mortuary.

I received a call from the crew who'd taken him in.

'Do you have the phone number the rugby club used to call 999?' they asked. 'The patient didn't make it, and no one travelled with him. We only know his first name. Somehow we need to get a message to his relatives. I know we could ask the patient with the leg injury, but ...'

She tailed off, but I knew exactly what she was thinking. Broken-leg guy had been through enough for now. I gave her

the number of the rugby club, thinking of that poor man's family
sitting at home waiting for him to come home from his match, dinner on the table, waiting and waiting until finally they received
*that* phone call. I was grateful that, while this job involves lots
of unenviable tasks, breaking the news to relatives isn't one of
them.

# All Change

12 February 2007

I'm being moved! Apparently my new position as allocator comes with a new desk and new colleagues. It's a bit of a shock – I thought I'd be able to stay here on the south-east, as they are short of an allocator anyway, but apparently the north-east on C Watch are even more in need of allocators. So it will be goodbye to Jenny and Snowy and to Sally and the other regulars and all the ambulance crews that I have come to know and love, and hello to a whole new desk!

My last shift here is next week – a night, on 15 February. I am also working on Valentine's Day. I'm not sorry that I am working on Valentine's Day. Going out somewhere and being surrounded by yucky happy couples who work sensible shifts and actually have time for a functional relationship is not my idea of fun!

# Valentine's Day

15 February 2007

I thought I knew what I was going to tell you about Valentine's Day. I was going to make some self-deprecating jokes about being a saddo singleton who hasn't had so much as a sniff of a boyfriend since breaking up with Alan, and who probably puts everyone off by wearing a horrible green uniform and living in a haunted flat. Then I would move on to some tales about rowing couples falling out over their Valentine's flowers and conclude that maybe it was best to be single and spend Valentine's night at work after all.

But then something happened that made me forget all about the shoddy rigmarole of Valentine's Day. Something awful and unforgettable. Something that would prove to be my biggest challenge to date.

Just after 8 p.m. we had a call from a neighbouring ambulance service. They'd gone to a call just outside London and the patient was a member of our staff – a paramedic from my sector – and they wanted one of our managers to attend. We sent the manager, and half an hour later he was on the phone. It turned out the paramedic in question had died suddenly at home. And now he had the unenviable task of breaking the news to her colleagues.

As the allocator in charge of the desk that night it was my job to stand down every single crew from three ambulance stations. This was while juggling a screen full of calls – the majority of which were, luckily, a load of utter rubbish. Every time an ambulance crew finished a job, I had to send them to the ambulance station where the deceased paramedic had worked to talk to the manager. Of course, the crews were totally confused as to why they were being sent there in the middle of a busy night shift when there were calls waiting. Most assumed they'd done something wrong. Others thought there had been some kind of major incident. Some started moaning about going there and saying they needed fuel or blankets. Of course, I couldn't say anything other than, 'It'll be explained when you get there' or, if really pressed, 'It's a staff issue.' The whole sense of knowing something they didn't know, and of withholding horrible news, made me feel really uneasy. I imagined all the crews piling into the ambulance station and wondering why there were so many ambulances there, then entering the mess room and finding their colleagues in tears and the poor manager having to explain yet again what had happened.

For the next hour or two we heard nothing from the ambulance station and the screen continued to fill up with calls, which I tried my hardest to cover with ambulances from other parts of the sector.

'Another call in Bromley?' complained a Beckenham crew. 'Where are all the Bromleys tonight?'

I told the crews rather ambiguously that there was a 'serious staffing issue in the Bromley area' and after a while they stopped asking.

Then my phone rang. It was Cheryl from New Addington, a jolly girl who only minutes ago I'd been having some friendly banter with about hospital transfers and LAS protocols. Now she was in tears.

'I've just heard about … Bromley …' she sniffed. 'I was bridesmaid at her wedding … I'm going to have to go off the road …'

Because Cheryl worked at New Addington, which is part of a different complex from Bromley, she hadn't been stood down and had found out on the grapevine when she'd bumped into another crew at hospital. Poor Cheryl. I sent her and her crewmate up to Bromley with the rest of them.

Around 1 a.m. the crews started to leave Bromley. They were all in a very difficult position because ordinarily a crew would be allowed to go home automatically after receiving bad news like this, but because there were at least twenty crews affected, if they all went home, the calls would never be covered (I already had thirty waiting) and patients could die. We let each crew choose for themselves whether they wanted to stay or go. Only two crews opted to go. The rest, including Cheryl, worked on. I was very grateful to them for doing so – it must have been so difficult, and I could hear how upset they were in their voices every time I spoke to them. It was seriously awful. I really felt for them, but there was nothing I could do except repeatedly offer to let them go home. But they all insisted on staying. They knew what could happen if they didn't.

As my last shift as a lowly Emergency Medical Dispatcher drew to a close, I thought about the important lesson that I'd learnt and that I would remember throughout the coming years as an allocator. The attitude that those crews had shown in the face of the death of their colleague was what keeps this service running. To help others, you have to forget your fears and your own personal tribulations so you can put others first. No one does that more than the ambulance crews, and it's an honour for me to be their allocator and to assist them in doing their jobs. I'm going to miss taking calls, but I'm really looking forward to being in charge of my new desk and meeting my new colleagues. I've had such an amazing experience over the last three years – who'd have thought this job would be so right for me? I'm almost glad that my attempts at learning to drive were so hopeless, because if I'd become a paramedic I would never have reached this stage. There's a whole fascinating world behind the scenes of the London Ambulance Service, and there's still so much for me to learn.

# Epilogue

# The Ten Commandments
## of Dialling 999

If you've learnt anything from reading this book, I hope it's how to make a good 999 call. But just in case you ever need a reminder, here are my Ten Commandments.

1. *Know thy Address.*
   Make sure you have a full street name, house number, area name and postal district, and any important information and landmarks which might help us find the address. If this isn't possible, call from a telephone box or other landline (ask in a shop or knock on someone's door) – we can trace the call. We can't trace the exact location of a mobile phone.

2. *Know thy Problem.*
   We get loads of calls from receptionists and security guards who have been asked to get an ambulance for someone else without being told what is happening. An ambulance is unlikely to be dispatched until they've told us what the problem is because we can't categorize the call and don't know what to dispatch.

3. *Stay With thy Patient.*
   You'll need to answer a few questions about the patient and possibly perform a bit of first aid, so it really helps if the person who is calling is sitting right next to the patient.

4. *Thou Shalt Not Waffle.*
   Give clear, concise answers to questions and don't be scared to say 'I don't know' if you don't know! Now is not the time to give the patient's entire life story.

5. *Trust thy Call Taker.*
   When I was a call taker, I used to spend about half an hour a day listening to callers 'helpfully' telling me things such

as: It's an emergency! You'd better get here fast! Stop asking questions and just send the ambulance. You could send one from Woolwich Ambulance Station, it's just around the corner. I think you're going to need the fire brigade too. Tell them to drive fast! Hurry up! Etc. Remember that we have been taking these calls day in, day out – for years. We don't need you to tell us how to do our job.

6. *Keep a Civil Tongue in thy Head.*
Yes, we know you're panicking, but really, there's no need to be rude. Tell the call taker she's an effing moron once too often and the blue flashing lights you see next will be attached to a police car!

7. *Thou Shalt Not Hang up Until Thou Art Told.*
On TV 999 calls are over in seconds. In real life you will be on the phone for approximately two to three minutes, or until the ambulance arrives. Don't hang up until the call taker says you can. Remember that the length of the call has absolutely no bearing on how long the ambulance will take to arrive, and that what the call taker is telling you is important.

8. *Keep thy Phone Switched On.*
Or give an alternative number. We often need to call people back for more information.

9. *Meet thy Ambulance.*
If you have a spare person at the scene, get them to stand in the middle of the road and do an impression of a windmill. The location may be obvious to you, but it is not always obvious to the ambulance crew – and while ambulance crews are usually local, this isn't always the case.

10. *Know thy First Aid.*
We can give you instructions over the phone, but don't wait until you are kneeling over a comatose relative to learn CPR. Ask your employer or St John Ambulance about going on a first-aid course.

# Glossary

A&E      Accident and Emergency department (in a hospital). Where the ambulance takes you.

Amber Calls      See 'Cat B Calls'.

AMPDS      Advance Medical Priority Dispatch System – the software which tells EMDs what to ask and what instructions to give.

BBA      Born Before Arrival. When someone decides to give birth either in the back of the ambulance or at home with the assistance of an EMD.

Blue Call      A pre-alert placed by an ambulance crew to a hospital via Control, notifying them that they are bringing in a seriously ill patient on blue lights.

Blued In      Taken to hospital by ambulance on blue lights. Means patient is not in a good way.

Cat A Calls      The most serious, life-threatening calls, assuming AMPDS has done its job and the caller has been truthful. Also known as 'red calls'.

Cat B Calls      Serious but not immediately life-threatening calls. Also known as 'amber calls'.

Cat C Calls      Calls that are neither serious nor immediately life-threatening. Also known as 'green calls'.

| | |
|---|---|
| *CTA* | Clinical Telephone Advice. A bunch of paramedics/EMTs who ring back green calls and try to find the most appropriate way of dealing with them, which often does not involve an ambulance. Formerly known as TAS (Telephone Advice Service). |
| *DSO* | Duty Station Officer – ambulance crews' manager. |
| *EMD* | Emergency Medical Dispatcher. Me. |
| *Emergency Operator* | The person who says 'Emergency, which service please?' and then puts you through to us. Works for telephone company, not emergency services. |
| *EMT* | Emergency Medical Technician. Like a paramedic, but not yet trained to do a few key things, mainly giving intravenous drugs. |
| *EOC* | Emergency Operations Centre. Otherwise known as 'the control room'. |
| *FRU* | First Response Unit or Fast Response Unit. An ambulance car staffed by one paramedic or EMT, used to reach the most serious calls as quickly as possible. |
| *GB* | General Broadcast. A broadcast on the ambulance radio aimed at all ambulances, usually 'advertising' a call that we want someone to cover. |
| *Green Calls* | See 'Cat C Calls'. |
| *Green Truck* | An ambulance with basic equipment staffed by technicians with less training. Designed to free up ordinary ambulances for life-threatening calls |

without detriment to less serious calls. They are not actually green – they are so called because they go to green calls.

HEMS        Helicopter Emergency Medical Service. Big red helicopter with doctor and paramedic on board that goes to the most serious trauma calls.

LAS         London Ambulance Service

Maternataxi  Misuse of ambulance system as a free ride to hospital by a woman in the early stages of labour with no medical emergency.

MDT         Mobile Data Terminal – the computer in the ambulance which tells the ambulance crew where and what they are going to and how to get there.

MPS         Metropolitan Police Service – London police force.

One Under    Person under a train.

Paramedic    Green-clad ambulance medic. Not to be called 'ambulance driver'.

Purple       Dead.

Purple Plus  Very obviously dead.

Red Calls    See 'Cat A Calls'.

Suspended    In cardiac arrest. Not dead *yet*.

UOC         Urgent Operations Centre – smaller control room upstairs that deals with lower-priority calls and looks after CTA and Green Trucks.

# Acknowledgements

Thanks to:

Jenny Lord, Juliet Annan, Shân Morley Jones and the fantastic Penguin sales, marketing and publicity teams for seeing the potential to turn *Nee Naw* from blog to book and for always being on hand to help me along the way.

Isabel White, my agent, for huge amounts of help and patience while introducing me to the world of publishing.

Steven Thurgood for hosting the *Nee Naw* site free of charge over the last four years. I suspect you didn't realize quite how much traffic it would get when you offered.

Eddie Johnson for the *Nee Naw* site design, and incredible patience when finding the perfect shades of green and yellow for the background.

All my friends for believing in me and encouraging me to unleash *Nee Naw* on to the general public. Particular thanks to C. J. Lines (Rattler) and Ollie Redfern for your invaluable feedback on my writing. Special mention to Clay Young (The American) for providing just the right level of distraction while I slaved over this book.

My mother, for ongoing generalized motherly services, taking me on holiday and buying me cocktails.

All the readers of *Nee Naw*, especially Tom Reynolds and his inspirational blog, *Random Acts of Reality*.

Everyone at the London Ambulance Service Communications Department and in Management, especially Tim Edmonds, for allowing me to keep my blog and to write this book, and for providing guidance without censorship.

All my colleagues at Nee Naw Control, especially Ange, G and Nikki on the east central and Jackie, Janice and Frosty on the north-east. Percy Pigs to all of you!

All the crews who have taken me out on observation days, especially Andy McCall of Putney. I learnt so much and it was a pleasure to help carry your oxygen cylinders.

The patients, the 999 callers and – most of all – the ambulance crews. Without you I wouldn't have a job. You make it all worthwhile. Thank you.

# MARINA LEWYCKA

## WE ARE ALL MADE OF GLUE

Georgie Sinclair's life is coming unstuck. Her husband's left her. Her son's obsessed with the End of the World. And now her elderly neighbour Mrs Shapiro has decided they are related.

Or so the hospital informs her when Mrs Shapiro has an accident and names Georgie next of kin. This, however, is not a case of a quick ward visit: Mrs Shapiro has a large rickety house full of stinky cats that needs looking after that a pair of estate agents seem intent on swindling from her. Plus there are the 'Uselesses' trying to repair it (uselessly). Then there's the social worker who wants to put her in a nursing home. Not to mention some letters that point to a mysterious, painful past.

As Georgie tries her best to put Mrs Shapiro's life back together somehow she must stop her own from falling apart . . .

'Vibrant dialogue, a family in meltdown, a clash of cultures and wonderful cast of expertly observed characters. Pure laugh-out-loud social comedy' *Daily Mail*

'Hilarious. A big-hearted confection of the comic and the poignant'
*Literary Review*

'A big, bustling novel, told with enthusiasm by a narrator who is warm, winningly disaster-prone and, crucially, believable' *Spectator*

# ZOË HELLER

**THE BELIEVERS**

When Audrey makes a devastating discovery about her husband, New York radical lawyer Joel Litvinoff, she is forced to re-examine everything she thought she knew about their forty-year marriage. Joel's children will have to deal with this unsettling secret themselves, but meanwhile, they are trying to cope with their own dilemmas.

Rosa, beautiful, disillusioned revolutionary, is grappling with a new-found attachment to Orthodox Judaism. Unhappily married Karla is falling in love with an unlikely suitor at the hospital where she works. Adopted brother Lenny is back on drugs again.

In the course of battling their own demons and each other, every member of the family is called upon to decide what – if anything – they still believe in.

'Astonishingly well-observed and stunningly written, a subtle, funny family farce…in its thundering confidence, *The Believers* is the work of a writer at the top of her game' *Guardian*

'One of the outstanding novels of the year…funny and elegant' Peter Kemp, *Sunday Times*

'Profoundly satisfying. No other novel would readily stand in its stead…pulses with thematic and intellectual content…Heller's prose is clean, warm and smart' Lionel Shriver, *Daily Telegraph*

# KATHRYN STOCKETT

**THE HELP**

Enter a vanished and unjust world: Jackson, Mississippi, 1962. Where black maids raise white children, but aren't trusted not to steal the silver...

There's Aibileen, raising her seventeenth white child and nursing the hurt caused by her own son's tragic death; Minny, whose cooking is nearly as sassy as her tongue; and white Miss Skeeter, home from College, who wants to know why her beloved maid has disappeared.

Skeeter, Aibileen and Minny. No one would believe they'd be friends; fewer still would tolerate it. But as each woman finds the courage to cross boundaries, they come to depend and rely upon one another. Each is in a search of a truth. And together they have an extraordinary story to tell...

'Outstanding, immensely funny, very compelling, brilliant' *Daily Telegraph*

'The other side of *Gone with the Wind* – and just as unputdownable' *Sunday Times*

'A laugh-out-loud, vociferously angry must-read' *Marie Claire*

# BICH MINH NGUYEN

## SHORT GIRLS

Linny and Van Luong are two second generation Vietnamese immigrant sisters from the American Midwest. Linny, the youngest, is pretty and popular but trapped in a cycle of dead-end jobs and hopeless affairs. Van, plain and socially awkward, is an overachieving immigration lawyer with a seemingly picture-perfect marriage. The sisters have been locked in a relationship of mutual disdain for as long as they can remember.

When their eccentric elderly father, inventor of the 'Luong Arm' (a gadget to help short people reach objects in high places), finally decides to take the oath for American citizenship in order to compete in an *American Idol*-style reality show for inventors, the sisters must return to their childhood home to plan a party to celebrate the decision that took thirty years to make. As they navigate their secrets, silences and all that has seemed out of reach to them for so long, Van and Linny realize that they are not so different from each other after all ...

'Loaded with tender charm and wry, lightly observed insights, this universal story embraces universal themes of family and belonging, as well as offering a glimpse of second-generation immigrant lives' *Daily Mail*

'Nguyen is an amusing observer of assimilation angst...this gentle-comedy of inter-generational strife is a polished and poised affair' *Independent*

'A well-structured, smoothly pleasurable read' *Guardian*

# JUDITH O'REILLY

---

## WIFE IN THE NORTH

350 miles from home, three young children and one very absent husband …

Maybe hormones ate her brain. How else did Judith's husband persuade her to give up her career and move from her beloved London to Northumberland with two toddlers in tow?

Pregnant with number three, Judith is about to discover that there are one or two things about life in the country that no one told her about: that she'd be making friends with people who believe in the four horsemen of the apocalypse; that running out of petrol could be a near-death experience; and that the closest thing to an ethnic minority would be a redhead.

Judith tries to do that simple thing that women do, make hers a happy family. A family that might live happily ever after. Possibly even up North …

'Funny, poignant and beautifully written' Lisa Jewell

'I howled with laughter, tears of recognition at every page' Jenny Colgan

'Genuinely funny and genuinely moving' Jane Fallon

---

# *He just wanted a decent book to read ...*

Not too much to ask, is it? It was in 1935 when Allen Lane, Managing Director of Bodley Head Publishers, stood on a platform at Exeter railway station looking for something good to read on his journey back to London. His choice was limited to popular magazines and poor-quality paperbacks – the same choice faced every day by the vast majority of readers, few of whom could afford hardbacks. Lane's disappointment and subsequent anger at the range of books generally available led him to found a company – and change the world.

*'We believed in the existence in this country of a vast reading public for intelligent books at a low price, and staked everything on it'*
**Sir Allen Lane, 1902–1970, founder of Penguin Books**

The quality paperback had arrived – and not just in bookshops. Lane was adamant that his Penguins should appear in chain stores and tobacconists, and should cost no more than a packet of cigarettes.

Reading habits (and cigarette prices) have changed since 1935, but Penguin still believes in publishing the best books for everybody to enjoy. We still believe that good design costs no more than bad design, and we still believe that quality books published passionately and responsibly make the world a better place.

So wherever you see the little bird – whether it's on a piece of prize-winning literary fiction or a celebrity autobiography, political tour de force or historical masterpiece, a serial-killer thriller, reference book, world classic or a piece of pure escapism – you can bet that it represents the very best that the genre has to offer.

**Whatever you like to read – trust Penguin.**